THE GREEN COFFEE BEAN
QUICK WEIGHT LOSS DIET

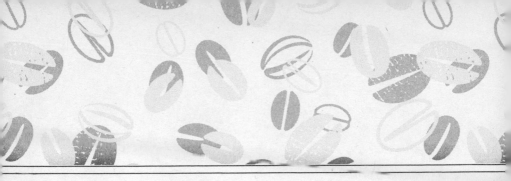

THE GREEN COFFEE BEAN

QUICK WEIGHT LOSS DIET

LESLIE PEPPER

FOREWORD BY STEVEN V. JOYAL, M.D.

A LYNN SONBERG BOOK

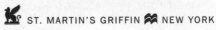

ST. MARTIN'S GRIFFIN ☂ NEW YORK

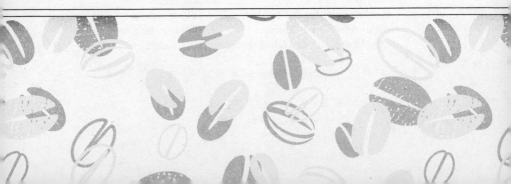

ISBN 978-1-250-04314-6 (trade paperback)
ISBN 978-1-4668-4124-6 (e-book)

St. Martin's Griffin books may be purchased for educational,
business, or promotional use. For information on bulk
purchases, please contact Macmillan Corporate and
Premium Sales Department at 1-800-221-7945 extension
5442 or write specialmarkets@macmillan.com.

First Edition: May 2013

10 9 8 7 6 5 4 3 2 1

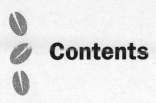

Contents

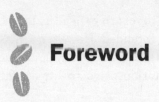

Foreword

During my career in medicine I've had the privilege of treating patients in private practice and academia, working with world-class scientists, leading complex pharmaceutical development projects, and guiding the integration of nutritional science into practical solutions for health and wellness. All of these experiences have helped shape my philosophy toward evidence-based approaches for helping people achieve optimal health.

In particular, I'm keenly interested in health concerns surrounding type 2 diabetes and obesity.

Green coffee is a natural nutritional product with very interesting implications for metabolic health. My experiences in pharmaceutical development, including being responsible for global drug development for metabolic conditions including type 2 diabetes and obesity, and now as chief medical officer for Life Extension, an organization dedicated to helping people live healthier, longer lives, has convinced me of the important role that nutrition plays in achieving optimal health. In addition to your level of physical activity, diet is the other major component of your lifestyle that has an enormous impact on your health.

However, no one—and I mean *no one*—consistently consumes a perfect diet. In today's world we are bombarded by advertising focused upon micronutrient-poor, calorically dense, cheap food. Literally an entire multibillion-dollar, multinational industry exists with the sole focus of determining how best to chemically modify unhealthy processed food in order to make that food *irresistible* to you.

We desperately need to return to healthy foods, minimally processed, the way nature intended. However, I'm a realist, too, and recognize that since no one consistently consumes a perfect diet, nutritional supplementation plays an important, vitally critical role in optimal health.

In several published, peer-reviewed scientific studies, green bean coffee extract, a natural product, has demonstrated intriguing, beneficial effects on a variety of metabolic health concerns, including blood sugar (blood glucose) as well as body weight.

Green coffee bean extract contains a variety of beneficial ingredients; however, for the purpose of simplicity, we'll focus upon just one, chlorogenic acid. This important active ingredient in green coffee bean extract works in several ways to support a healthy body weight and blood sugar levels. For example, chlorogenic acid inhibits the activity of a liver enzyme called glucose-6-phosphatase, which releases glucose from the liver into the bloodstream; over the long term, when blood sugar levels are too high, damage occurs to your blood vessels, your nerves, your eyes, and your kidneys.

As another example, chlorogenic acid helps support the metabolism of fat in the liver, which is important for healthy body weight management. Another beneficial effect of chlorogenic acid is that the compound helps slow down the rapid absorption of sugar from the digestive tract, helping to reduce wild spikes in blood sugar in response to a meal rich in excess carbohydrate (sugar, starch).

There are no "magic pills" that effortlessly melt excess body fat, and anyone who promises such an elixir should be greeted with a healthy dose of skepticism. Lifestyle modifications will always remain important: following a healthy diet, engaging in regular physical exercise, and managing stress (stress can cause blood sugar levels to rise) are crucial steps everyone needs to take for optimal health and healthy body weight management.

But no one consistently consumes a perfect diet. Further, I understand that making healthy lifestyle changes while trying to maintain a household, raise children, have a successful career, and cope with the countless little stressors and aggravations of daily life can be very challenging!

For many people, green coffee bean extract may help make the goals of healthier blood sugar levels and weight management a bit easier, and more rapidly *achievable*.

Leslie Pepper has written an excellent, practical guide which explains everything you need to know about utilizing this interesting new supplement to support your health.

—*Steven V. Joyal, M.D.*
April 2013

CHAPTER 1

A Different Kind of Diet

How many times have you tried to lose weight? Ten times? Twenty times? Maybe even a hundred times? Each of those times, you struggled, you starved, and you ended up right back where you started. You may have even ended up heavier than you were when you began. Why? Because diets based on deprivation don't work and, let's face it, most diets are all about deprivation. They've got boring and denial built right into them. They take away your freedom of choice—a recipe for disaster.

Even if you do manage to stay with carrot sticks and celery stalks for a while, you'll eventually end up taking a few spoonfuls of Ben & Jerry's. Then you'll feel guilty and ashamed and probably end up devouring the entire pint. And then you'll go back to deprivation and end up hungry and miserable.

Drastically reducing the amount of food you take in while cutting out all your favorite treats simply isn't sustainable for most people. You cannot eat that way for any length of time. Sooner or later, you go right back to eating exactly the way you did before. Even worse, you'll eat more, because you've been missing all your favorite foods for the time you were on that diet.

Now, what if we said you could lose weight without feeling deprived? Yes, it sounds too good to be true, but according to research published in a respected scientific journal, it's 100 percent genuine. We'll go into the research in more detail later, but to give you a taste (pun intended): a breakthrough study found that participants who took a supplement containing green coffee bean extract lost an average of 17 pounds in twenty-two weeks. *Without changing the way they ate.*

Researchers attribute the result to a plant compound found in the unroasted coffee bean called chlorogenic acid. This phytonutrient may have some effect on reducing blood glucose absorption, which in turn helps keep weight down. Even better news: you don't have to be part of a research study in order to get the benefits of green coffee bean extract. The supplement is available in stores nationwide.

If you want to duplicate the results of this study, you can do so simply by reading and following the instructions in chapters 2 and 3 in this book. In those chapters we'll explain the science of why and how the supplement works, and we'll give you all the information you need to know about buying and taking a supplement. According to the study, you don't have to change your diet in order to lose weight slowly with the green coffee bean extract. By tamping down the insulin response, the supplement, all by itself, will do the work for you.

However, that's not what makes this book special and not what we'd recommend. We're going to do one better and provide you with an eating and exercise plan that's based not on deprivation but actually on the exact opposite. Our diet is based on gratification. You will be able to eat plenty of food—enough so that you'll never feel hungry and grouchy. Plus, you'll be able to treat yourself to your favorite foods—and still lose weight. This nondeprivation diet will set you on the road to lifelong slimness and health. Since you'll never feel like you're missing anything, this is a diet you can stay on for good. No yo-yoing back and forth between dress sizes. This time when you lose the weight, it will stay off.

But before we tell you more about why this diet will work for you, let's take a moment to see why so many of us struggle to reach our ideal weight.

Overweight and obesity among adults 20 years of age and over

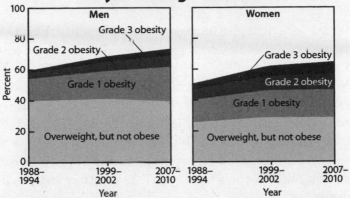

NOTE: Overweight but not obese is body mass index (BMI) greater than or equal to 25 but less than 30; grade 1 obesity is BMI greater than or equal to 30 but less than 35; grade 2 obesity is BMI greater than or equal to 35 but less than 40; grade 3 obesity is BMI greater than or equal to 40.
SOURCE: CDC/NCHS, *Health, United States, 2011*, Figure 11. Data from the National Health and Nutrition Examination Survey.

A WIDESPREAD (AHEM) PROBLEM

If you're trying to lose weight, and have been for a while, you're not alone in your plight. During the past twenty years, the scales in this country have been tipping, and not in our favor. According to the Centers for Disease Control and Prevention (CDC), a staggering one third of the adults in the United States are overweight.

DANGEROUS DEVELOPMENTS

Sure, we want to lose weight to look good. But being overweight is more than just a matter of aesthetics. Obesity-related conditions include some of the leading causes of preventable death. They include:

- Heart disease
- Stroke

- Type 2 diabetes
- Certain types of cancers

Being overweight also increases your risk for high blood pressure, high blood cholesterol, gallbladder disease, sleep apnea, and osteoarthritis.

But there is good news: with even a small amount of weight loss, blood cholesterol will come down, blood pressure will begin to normalize, and blood sugar will improve. Your risk of having a heart attack or a stroke will decrease and you'll reduce your risk of developing type 2 diabetes. Not only will you look better when you take off the weight, you'll feel better, and you'll be healthier.

 HOW DID WE GET HERE?

Our weight is climbing steadily, and right now there's no end in sight. Unfortunately, our modern culture seems to be working against us. Technology has made our lives infinitely easier, and also easier for us to get fat. We've engineered almost all physical activity out of our lives; we no longer have to hunt for our food—it's delivered right to our cars at a very affordable price. The food we eat is highly processed and full of sugar, salt, and fat. We spend hours in front of screens—computer, television, and handheld—never having to get up to change a channel or even deliver a fax. According to the Centers for Disease Control and Prevention, less than half of all adults meet the Physical Activity Guidelines set by the government. No wonder we're a nation of fatties.

WHY THE GREEN COFFEE BEAN EXTRACT DIET?

You may be thinking to yourself, *Why another diet book?* You've tried every diet under the sun, and you've been here many times. Why should this diet be any different?

What you haven't had is the help of a supplement called green coffee bean extract. As we mentioned earlier, a study found that people who took a supplement containing green coffee bean extract lost an average of 17 pounds in twenty-two weeks without changing the way they ate. So you *can* lose weight without doing anything differently. That's great news, but we are going to offer you so much more.

As we've already mentioned, the problem with so many diets is that they're all about deprivation—what you *can't* eat. What's different about the green coffee bean extract diet is it's about what you *can* eat. Instead of focusing on the foods to take *out* of your diet, this meal plan focuses on what you can add *in*. This diet is all about being healthy—adding in plenty of good-for-you foods that fill you up without adding extra empty calories. Foods high in fiber, protein, vitamins and minerals, and low in saturated fat. When eating in this nutritionally balanced way, you'll feel more energetic, so you'll want to continue to eat this way even without seeing the numbers on the scale drop. But don't worry—you *will* see those numbers go down. And when you do, you'll want to keep going with our healthy weight-loss plan.

On this diet, we focus on:

- **VOLUME:** The core concept of the green coffee bean extract diet is that you get to eat a lot of food without gaining weight. We'll show you how to choose the right foods— foods that are known as high-volume foods, foods that take up a lot of room on the plate, but have very few calories; foods that have a lot of air and water, which tricks your senses into thinking you've eaten more than you actually have; and foods that are high in fiber, which add a lot of heft and health to food. We'll show you that when you eat foods that have fewer calories per bite, your portion size grows but your overall calorie count stays the same.

- **SATISFACTION:** Our meal plans, should you choose to follow them, provide three meals and two snacks per day. We'll show you how to always make sure you eat enough healthy, high-volume, low-calorie foods to avoid hunger. You'll be given tons of food choices that you can add to your diet so you'll never ever feel your stomach growling. On this diet you won't have to starve yourself to lose weight. In fact, if you feel a rumble in your stomach, that's a sign that you're not eating enough.

- **TREATING YOURSELF:** On our diet you'll learn the difference between a snack and a treat. A snack is a small amount of food to satisfy your hunger in between meals. A treat is something a bit more indulgent—a small scoop of frozen yogurt, a few cookies, a piece of dark chocolate— that you might enjoy once in a while. On this diet you're allowed to have treats, which will help to keep you on track.

Stella, forty-one years old, tall, brunette, with big blue eyes, and a dazzling grin, came from a family of overeaters. In her home growing up, there was always a ton of food on the table. Steaks, chicken, and pork chops were accompanied by thick sauces and carbohydrates piled high. Potatoes with butter and sour cream, pasta with Alfredo sauce, and French fries were staples in Stella's house. And although her mother usually made some sort of vegetable to go with dinner—broccoli, carrots, or cauliflower— Stella and her brother and sister would pour heaps of cheese sauce on top. So it's no surprise that Stella overate and became overweight.

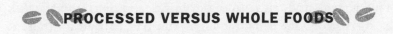 PROCESSED VERSUS WHOLE FOODS

It's important to know the difference between a product derived from many ingredients to look and taste like food . . . and real food. When you eat one-ingredient whole foods you're feeding your body health-supporting nutrition that makes you feel satisfied without those awful cravings. (Think fruits, vegetables, nuts, lean proteins— how many ingredients? Just one!) Processed foods, one the other hand, may provide instant gratification, but they don't give your body sustenance, are loaded with chemicals and preservatives, and in the end, make you feel pretty lousy. A simple trick: look at the label and pay attention to the number of ingredients. If there's a long list of words you can't pronounce, better to stay away.

After her father died of a heart attack in his fifties, Stella's weight ballooned even more. "I was so depressed about my dad, and it didn't even occur to me that I could be on the same path—to an early death," she says. "Or, maybe I was just in complete denial." By her thirtieth birthday, Stella's weight topped 175 pounds. It wasn't until her mother died of complications due to type 2 diabetes that Stella realized she needed to lose the weight. "It finally hit me. I was going to die unless I did something. And fast," Stella says.

Stella went to her doctor, who pointed her to a local diet center that sold packaged meals. Stella signed up, and although she was hungry and cranky every day, within two weeks she'd dropped six pounds. She was so thrilled to see the numbers on that scale drop, she almost didn't even mind the tasteless food and the constant empty pit in her stomach.

That is, until the scale slowed down. By week five, she began to really miss her favorite foods. She couldn't get the image of a juicy steak and fries out of her mind, and by the sixth week of starvation, she'd had enough. She had to find a different way.

She knew the packaged-food diet wouldn't work for her because she felt so deprived. She'd heard about the green coffee bean extract diet, so she decided to give it a try. She was skeptical, but invested in a month's supply of green coffee extract. At first, she didn't change anything in her diet, yet she managed to take off two pounds in three weeks. "Hey, maybe there is something to this," she thought, and she headed to the store to fill her cart with high-volume fruits and vegetables, lots of fiber-filled foods, and lean cuts of meat. "I figured if the supplement could help me lose weight slowly, maybe if I actually followed the diet, I'd lose weight quicker."

And lose weight quickly she did—without feeling even one hunger pang. "I learned that for the same number of calories in a measly little portion of broccoli with cheese sauce, I could eat a whole huge plate of broccoli, which actually, if you put a little olive oil, lemon juice, and ginger on it, tasted delicious. I knew that pouring the cheese sauce on the broccoli wouldn't give me enough to fill me up, so I didn't bother with it anymore." Well, most of the time. Two meals a week, Stella allowed herself license to eat whatever she wanted . . . without binge eating of course. Then she'd go back to following the healthy menu plan she'd read in the book.

She started experimenting with foreign foods and spices, and she continued to slim down until she reached her goal weight, without feeling the least bit deprived. "The diet was easy because I got to eat all my favorite foods, and I never felt hungry." The best part? Stella shared her diet secrets with her brother and sister. Now they're on the green coffee bean extract diet, on their way to healthier lives, too!

Quiz: Do You Need This Diet?

Even if your weight is within the normal range, you may still want to think about following this plan. Take this quiz to see if you may be on your way to weighing too much.

Answer yes or no to the following questions:

1. Do you often skip breakfast?

   ☐ Yes　　　☐ No

2. Do you spend a lot of time sitting during the day?

   ☐ Yes　　　☐ No

3. Do you often think about food, and spend time planning around your meals?

   ☐ Yes　　　☐ No

4. Do you often do other things—watching television, reading, or driving—while you eat?

   ☐ Yes　　　☐ No

5. Do you eat food straight out of the package?

   ☐ Yes　　　☐ No

6. Do you eat food while standing at the counter?

   ☐ Yes　　　☐ No

7. Would you say you eat quickly?

   ☐ Yes　　　☐ No

8. Do you take big bites of food?

   ☐ Yes　　　☐ No

If you answered yes to more than two of these questions, you might want to think about your eating habits. Even if you're not overweight now, your routines make it likely that you'll get there.

In this chapter we've given you a glimpse of how our high-volume, nondeprivation diet can help you lose weight . . . and we hope you are intrigued enough to read on. In the next chapter we're going to explain how the chlorogenic acid in the supplement we've been talking about—green coffee bean extract—works in scientific terms to become your partner in weight loss. As many women and men have already discovered, green coffee bean extract can help you achieve the weight-loss goal you've wanted for years, the one that has eluded you until now.

Then, after you learn about the supplement, you'll be given the tools you need to lose the weight. You'll find tips and tricks on how to get and stay motivated. You'll get a detailed eating plan so you'll know exactly what to eat and how. You'll get recipes so you can eat according to our plan and you'll be given some exercise ideas to help you boost your weight loss even more. We'll also give you tools and techniques to help you through any setbacks you may experience along the way.

Nothing good in life comes with zero effort. But you'll be pleasantly surprised at how easy this weight-loss plan can be. This book and lifestyle plan will support you every step of this very important journey.

CHAPTER 2

Green Coffee Bean Extract: How and Why It Works

Ready to get started? In this chapter we're going to introduce you to the supplement we touched on before, green coffee bean extract. You're going to learn more about what it is, and why it can help you. You're going to learn about an antioxidant in the extract called chlorogenic acid, and how it battles not only obesity, but other health issues as well. And we're going to lay out all the science for you in a way that you can understand, even without a Ph.D. in chemistry.

You may not realize this, but the coffee beans you see in your local Starbucks bear no resemblance to what they look like starting out. Surprisingly enough, coffee beans are not actually beans at all; they just resemble them. In reality, they're seeds, or pits, found inside the red or purple fruit that's produced by a flowering shrub commonly referred to as a coffee tree. They grow in a band around the equator between the Tropics of Capricorn and Cancer, an area high in elevation and rich in volcanic soils.

When the coffee seeds are cultivated, they are stripped of the fruit (there's not much there and it's not very good to eat), soaked, rinsed, sorted, and dried. Then they're shipped green to factories around the world. The beans are then roasted to bring out the rich colors and bold flavors that we associate with coffee. Finally, they are ground and brewed, and end up in your mug, piping hot.

Coffee is chockful of chemicals, and actually contains over eight hundred different compounds, including caffeine, sucrose, cellulose, and one we'll talk about later in this chapter, chlorogenic acid, the key to the coffee bean extract's weight-reducing effect. But before we look at chlorogenic acid, let's take a look at coffee itself, and some of the many benefits you can get from it.

DEATH DEFIER

Researchers at the National Institutes of Health, along with the American Association of Retired People, looked at more than 400,000 people over a span of thirteen years. After adjusting for smoking and other factors, they found that the more coffee the subjects drank, the more likely they were to survive. And they found that beneficial effect applied to both caffeinated and decaffeinated coffee. Specifically, coffee drinking appeared to cut the risk of dying from heart disease, lung disease, strokes, injuries, accidents, diabetes, and infections.

DIABETES DESTROYER

A study published in the *Journal of the American Medical Association* reviewed nine studies on coffee and type 2 diabetes. Of more than 193,000 people, those who said they drank more than six or seven cups daily were 35 percent less likely to have type 2 diabetes than people who drank fewer than two cups daily. And the *Journal of Agricultural and Food Chemistry* reported that people who drank four or more cups of coffee daily had a 50 percent lower risk of type 2 diabetes. Each additional cup of coffee added another decrease in risk of almost seven percent.

BRAIN CHAMPION

In one study of 676 elderly people, coffee consumption was associated with significantly less cognitive decline over a ten-year time frame. Three cups a day were associated with the least cognitive decline, with a remarkable 4.3-times smaller level of decline in cognitive function compared to noncoffee drinkers. Another study found that out of 1,400 people followed for about twenty years, those who reported drinking three to five cups of coffee daily were 65 percent less likely to develop dementia and Alzheimer's disease, compared with nondrinkers or occasional coffee drinkers.

GETTING TO GREEN COFFEE BEAN EXTRACT

So you see, coffee has its perks. And while caffeine can take credit for many of those perks, another compound found in coffee boosts your health as well. Much of coffee's bitter taste comes from a polyphenol known as chlorogenic acid, and concentrations in a cup of brewed coffee vary widely. Levels depend on roasting time and temperature, as well as the type of beans themselves. *Arabica* beans have lower levels than *Robusta*, for example.

Let's turn our attention again to the study we touched on in the previous chapter. Researchers found that a group of overweight or obese people who consumed coffee bean extract lost about 10 percent of their body weight. Sounds provocative, yes?

Joe Vinson, Ph.D., professor of chemistry at the University of Scranton, and his colleagues put sixteen overweight or obese people aged twenty-two to twenty-six years old through three phases during a twenty-two-week study. Each phase of the study lasted six weeks. During one phase, subjects were given a low daily dose of green bean coffee extract (700 mg). During another phase, they were given a higher dose of the extract (1,050 mg), and during a third phase they were given capsules containing a placebo (an inactive powder). Between each of the three phases there was a "wash-out" phase, in which participants took no pills at all.

It's important to note that the researchers used green coffee bean extract that contained 45.9 percent chlorogenic acid. This is an essential piece of information that you'll need when you shop for supplements since many of them will *not* contain a sufficient amount of the chlorogenic acid to help you lose weight. We'll give you detailed information on what to look for in a supplement in the next chapter.

Study Participants:	Age twenty-two to twenty-six, overweight or obese
Dosages of green coffee extract:	phase 1: 700 mg a day phase 2: 1050 mg a day phase 3: placebo
Diet before and during study:	Carbohydrate, fat, and protein intake remained about the same
Calorie intake:	Average calorie intake was 2400/day before and during study
Exercise:	Average 400 calories expended before and during study
Average weight loss:	seventeen pounds over course of twenty-two-week study

This type of study is called a crossover study, since each person took part in every phase of the study. In a crossover study, each person serves as his or her own control group, which improves the chances of getting an accurate result.

The participants were not told what to eat or how much they should eat throughout the study, though researchers did monitor their overall diet (number of calories, type of food eaten, etc.). Their calorie, carbohydrate, fat, and protein intakes stayed about the same during the study compared to those before the study began, with an average intake of about 2,400 calories per day. Exercise didn't change either, with each participant burning roughly 400 calories a day in physical activity.

What researchers found was this: Over the period of the twenty-two-week study, the participants lost an average of 17 pounds. This was an average of a 10.5 percent decrease in overall body weight and a 16 percent decrease in body fat. While that might not seem like a huge number, Vinson noted that the participants' weight loss might have been significantly faster had they received only the higher dose of the extract. Remember, all participants went through all phases of the study—so they received the placebo and the lower dose of green coffee bean extract for part of the study period, and no extract at all during the wash-out periods, all of which may have slowed down weight loss.

At a meeting of the American Chemical Society where Vinson presented his findings, he said, "Based on our results, taking multiple capsules of green coffee bean extract a day—while eating a low-fat, healthful diet and exercising regularly—appears to be a safe, effective, inexpensive way to lose weight."

So what is the compound in green coffee beans that makes them such fat fighters? Vinson does not believe it's the caffeine, but instead, he attributes the beneficial effect of green coffee beans to a plant chemical we mentioned earlier: chlorogenic acid.

HOW IT WORKS: CHLOROGENIC ACID
AND GLUCOSE METABOLISM

In order to understand how chlorogenic acid works to help you lose weight, you need to understand how glucose and the hormone insulin work together in the body. Hormones are complex molecules produced by the endocrine glands that control just about every aspect of how your body functions, including your mood, your interests, your libido, and your appetite. One of the key hormones involved in appetite is called insulin, produced by the pancreas, which the body uses to process glucose (sugar), and regulate your cravings for fat and carbohydrates. Insulin levels also have a hold on how you store calories, and whether or not you're able to lose weight on a certain diet.

After a meal, carbohydrates (which are sugars) are absorbed from the intestines into the bloodstream. When blood glucose rises, your pancreas responds by producing insulin, which clears the sugar out of the blood and into cells. Insulin causes excess sugar to be converted into fat for storage in the body. Over time, if you consume too many calories, the body stores those extra calories as body fat. And after a while, the body begins to lose its sensitivity to insulin, so it takes more and more insulin to regulate your blood sugar. This resistance to insulin is a major factor associated with full-blown type 2 diabetes.

Chlorogenic acid seems to put the brakes on the release of glucose into the bloodstream. It also appears to increase insulin sensitivity, and decrease the storage of both fat and carbohydrate. Chlorogenic acid inhibits *glucose-6-phosphatase,* a liver enzyme that liberates glucose in the liver to enter the blood. Excessive activity of this enzyme contributes to extra amounts of glucose released into the blood, contributing to after-meal blood-sugar spikes and increased blood glucose levels between meals. Chlorogenic acid also inhibits glucose absorption from the intestinal tract. Chlorogenic acid may also cause the liver to metabolize fat faster, making it a super-strength fat incinerator.

MORE THAN JUST WEIGHT LOSS

In addition to being a weight-loss aid, chlorogenic acid also acts as an antioxidant. An anti-what, you ask? In order to understand what an antioxidant is you first need to be familiar with free radicals. Think about what happens when you leave a sliced apple out for any length of time. It turns brown, right? That's a result of a natural process called oxidation, when a substance is exposed to oxygen and electrons from an atom or molecule are decreased.

Now imagine that sliced apple is the inside of your body; oxidation occurs there, too. When we convert food to energy inside the body, oxidation happens. We rust, so to speak. Additionally, recent research supports that exposure to certain things in the environment, such as tobacco smoke, unprotected sun, and radiation cause oxidation.

Inside the body, the process of oxidation generates a dangerous byproduct called free radicals—cells that are missing a critical molecule. Those cells seek to pair with other molecules to make up for the ones they're missing.

A DAMAGING SEARCH

When free radicals are on the hunt for an unpaired electron, they attack the nearest stable (or paired) molecule, stealing an electron and injuring the molecule in the process. While this initially stabilizes the free radical, the attacked molecule is now left with an unpaired electron, and it becomes a free radical itself, beginning a chain reaction during which thousands of free-radical reactions can occur within a few seconds. In time, DNA is damaged, the cell is mutated, and it grows and reproduces abnormally.

ANTIOXIDANTS TO THE RESCUE

The good news: Your body has its own superheroes called antioxidants, that prevent free radicals from damaging cells by stabilizing, or deactivating them before they attack. Think of those free radicals as bowling balls, coming down the lane and slamming around, knocking down all the pins. Antioxidants catch the balls before they're able to wreak any havoc. They stop the damage before it starts.

Free radicals may play a role in heart disease, cancer, and other diseases. While studies on chlorogenic acid are limited, we can assume that it has the same type of beneficial effect on the body as the antioxidants we're familiar with, such as vitamins A, C, and E, beta carotene, and lycopene.

There are interesting studies on chlorogenic acid that were done in several areas, including the following:

BLOOD PRESSURE

In one double-blind, placebo-controlled study of 117 men with mild hypertension, green coffee bean extract was given daily for one month at several different doses (46 mg, 93 mg, or 185 mg). After twenty-eight days, the two higher-dosage groups showed significant improvement in blood pressure as compared with the placebo. And the results seen were dose related. In other words, the higher the dosage, the greater the improvement, increasing the likelihood that the green coffee bean extract was the reason for improvement.

HEART CONDITIONS

Since chlorogenic acid acts as an antioxidant, it mops up destructive free-radical molecules, which can contribute to heart disease. Chlorogenic acid also appears to influence adenosine, a chemical that controls the rate at which nerves transmit messages. Studies have shown that chlorgenic acid increases the levels of adenosine by preventing its reabsorption in the body. Adenosine helps to dilate arteries, allowing more blood to flow through. This may help prevent heart muscle from being starved of blood, the cause of painful angina and heart attacks.

So, in this chapter you learned how green coffee bean extract can help you in your weight-loss journey, and you've heard about the exciting research done on it. It's a lot to understand, we know, but this information is important as you finally begin to lose weight, keep it off for good, feeling more satisfied and healthier than ever before. Now you've got the exciting research and we have explained what scientists think is going on in the body. Next, we'll tell you all you need to know when looking for and buying a supplement.

CHAPTER 3

What to Look for in a Supplement

Not all supplements are created equal. In this chapter we'll tell you what you need to know about them. You'll find out what the rules are surrounding supplements and what to look for in a green coffee bean extract supplement. We'll also give you some helpful hints about how to remember to take your green coffee bean capsule.

Remember the study done by Joe Vinson at the University of Scranton? He gave overweight or obese people two different dosages of green coffee bean extract plus a placebo over a twenty-two-week period and found that they lost an average of seventeen pounds without changing their diet. We're sure you'll want to replicate the study as closely possible, so let's look in a little more detail to the specifics used in the study.

The green coffee bean extract used in the Vinson study was provided by Applied Food Sciences in Austin, Texas, under the trade name GCA. GCA contains a green coffee bean extract standardized at 45.9 percent.

The study used two dosage levels of GCA, as well as a placebo. The high dose was 350 mg of GCA taken by mouth three times a day, (for a total of 1050 mg of GCA) and the low dose was 350 mg of GCA taken by mouth twice a day (for a total of 700 mg of GCA). Since many green coffee bean extract supplements come in 400 mg dosages, to best replicate the results of the study, take

400 mg of GCA, three times per day, thirty minutes before each meal.

RULES AND REGULATIONS

Because of this promising study, dozens of companies are now trying to cash in on the green coffee bean extract action. And you'd be wise to be wary and not believe the claims on every green coffee bean extract box. Green coffee bean extract is considered a dietary supplement, not a drug, and the rules for each are distinct.

A dietary supplement is defined by the Food and Drug Administration (FDA) as any product intended for ingestion as a supplement to the diet. This may include vitamins, minerals, herbs or other botanicals, amino acids, and substances such as enzymes. It's easy to spot a supplement because the law requires manufacturers to include the words "dietary supplement" on product labels.

Before 1994 dietary supplements were regulated the same as any food by the FDA and it was responsible for overseeing that their labeling was truthful. Things changed, however, in October of 1994, when the Dietary Supplement Health and Education Act (DSHEA) was signed into law by President Clinton. At the time, millions of consumers and manufacturers wanted dietary supplements to be available without prescriptions, and manufacturers wanted to be able to sell supplements with minimal regulations. So, DSHEA mandated that the FDA's job overseeing dietary supplements would begin only *after* the product enters the marketplace.

The bottom line? Be cautious when looking for a green coffee bean extract and do follow our advice in the section below. Some brands of green coffee bean extract do not specify the amount of chlorogenic acid that their supplements contain and others may not have accurate labeling.

WHAT TO LOOK FOR IN A SUPPLEMENT

Green coffee bean extract is not solely available in health-food stores. The supplement is sold in grocery, drug, and national discount chain stores, as well as through the Internet. Caveat emptor could not be more important when it comes to buying supplements, particularly when you're shopping on the Internet.

When looking for a green coffee bean extract supplement, always look at the list of ingredients. It should contain at least 45 percent chlorogenic acid extract, with no fillers and no artificial ingredients. Keep in mind, however, that a manufacturer could potentially skimp on an ingredient or even add chlorogenic acid compounds to a supplement without actually using green coffee bean extract. In addition to GCA (the trademarked green coffee bean extract owned by Applied Food Sciences that Vinson used in his study), Svetol is another reliable, trademarked green coffee bean extract.

ConsumerLab.com is an independent company providing test results and information to help consumers and health-care professionals identify the best quality health and nutrition products. The company tested several different green coffee bean extract products sold in the United States and analyzed their chemical constituents, checking for specific and total chlorogenic acid. Their entire report can be read at ConsumerLab.com, (you need to be a ConsumerLab.com member, $33/year to access reports covering more than a thousand vitamins and supplements). They found that four of the supplements they tested did not contain the expected amounts of chlorogenic acid—ranging from *no* detectable chlorogenic acid to 81 percent of the stated levels.

Tod Cooperman, M.D., president of ConsumerLab.com, did give us permission to share the following information: One of the eight supplements contained no detectable chlorogenic acid. Two of the brands that contained the stated quantities of chlorogenic acid, while not exceeding ConsumerLab's stringent

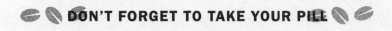

DON'T FORGET TO TAKE YOUR PILL

It's important to take your green coffee bean extract every day, thirty minutes before each meal. To help you remember:

- Take it at the same times every day so it becomes a habit. Couple it with a daily task, like brushing your teeth or eating your three meals.
- Set the alarm on your watch, cell phone, or BlackBerry to help you remember. Or sign up with a free service that sends an e-mail every day to remind you.
- Keep a chart, checklist, or calendar in a prominent place and mark when you've taken your green coffee bean extract.
- Use a day-of-the-week divided pillbox so you'll see exactly what you need to take and when.
- Put a picture of yourself in a bikini on the refrigerator with a sticky note, "Did you take your pill today?" (It will help you remember to take your pill *and* choose delicious healthy foods to eat!)
- Keep the bottle on the kitchen counter or by the sink so you remember to take it before each meal. Carry an extra bottle in your purse for dining out.
- Put a sticky note on your front door or by where you keep your keys asking yourself whether you've remembered your pills today.

criteria for lead or cadmium contamination were Life Extension Green Coffee Extract and Vitamin World Green Coffee Bean Extract.

Please keep in mind that there are many more brands available than ConsumerLab tested. For example, some other reliable

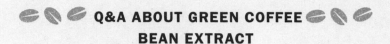

Q&A ABOUT GREEN COFFEE BEAN EXTRACT

Can green coffee bean extract really help me lose weight?
According to research published in *Diabetes, Metabolic Syndrome and Obesity*, yes. Researchers there gave a group of overweight or obese people various doses of green coffee bean extract, as well as a placebo, and the group lost about 10 percent of their body weight without changing their diet.

How does green coffee bean extract help you lose weight?
The researchers attribute the result to a compound called chlorogenic acid, which may tamp down the amount of glucose entering the bloodstream, which in turn reduces excess glucose from being converted into unsightly body fat.

How can I make sure the green bean coffee extract I buy contains chlorogenic acid?

brands include: NatureWise Svetol Green Coffee Bean Extract Ultra Pure with GCA Natural Weight Loss Supplement, and Pure Health Pure Green Coffee Bean Extract. If you see either GCA or Svetol on the ingredient label, you can be certain the extract contains at least 45 percent chlorogenic acid.

BE WARY OF THE WEB

Sometimes you can find inexpensive products on the Web, but when it comes to supplements, this is one time where it *does* pay to splurge. Lots of Web sites sell inexpensive supplements on the

Look at the list of ingredients. Green coffee bean extract contains chlorogenic acid if the ingredients list Green Coffee Bean extract, GCA (brand name), or Svetol (also a brand name). And make sure to only buy brands whose label says "contains 45 or 50 percent chlorogenic acid."

How much do I take?
Capsules will range in dosage. They can be 150 mg, 200 mg, 400 mg, 800 mg, etc. For best results, and to duplicate the dosages given in the study, take one 400 mg capsule thirty minutes before each meal and make sure the supplement you are taking contains at least 45 percent chlorogenic acid.

Who is green coffee bean extract right for?
Most healthy adults, over the age of eighteen can use green coffee bean extract. Women who are pregnant or breastfeeding should not take the supplement. This is not for children.

cheap, but you may not get what you expect. Anyone can create a pretty Web site with bells and whistles and easily claim they're operating out of the United States when they're really in a backyard garage in Bangladesh. If you purchase supplements from these rogue sites, there's no guarantee what you pay for is what you get. The product may have too much, too little, or even none of the active ingredient you need. While there are many Web sites that operate legally and offer convenience and privacy, there are just as many shady operations.

SOME SIGNS OF AN UNSAFE SITE:

- It advertises a supplement with unknown quality.
- The product is labeled primarily in a foreign language, or the Web site has misspelled words and has used poor grammar.
- It doesn't provide consumers with a way to contact the site by phone.
- It offers prices that are dramatically lower than its competitors.

While you know that you want to lose weight, you may be unconsciously sabotaging your efforts to do just that. The next chapter will help you sort that out and get you started on your way. Ready? Let's do it!

CHAPTER 4

Are You Ready to Lose Weight?

In the previous chapters, you learned all about a new weight-loss tool you can add to your arsenal. Green coffee bean extract can help you lose weight, even without changing your diet. And although you will probably lose weight simply by adding the extract into your day, we've got an even better idea for you.

How about changing the way you're eating as well, so you can fit into those skinny jeans even faster? We're not talking wilted lettuce leaves here; the plan we've created will help you achieve your weight-loss goal quickly and easily without deprivation. Yes, no more going hungry, no more saying no to delicious food choices, and no more disappointments when you step on the scale. We're going to teach you how to eat *more*, but weigh *less*.

But before we dive into the plan we've created, we first need to assess where your head is at. In this chapter we're going to figure out whether or not you're really ready to lose weight. We're also going to explore how much weight you should expect to lose and how quickly, and what to expect on the diet. We're also going to help you put some strategies for success into place so you're really ready to lose all the weight you want.

ARE YOU REALLY READY?

Tasha, twenty-nine, goes gung ho into every diet she starts. She clears out the pantry of junk and buys a month-long membership to a gym. And after three weeks of "perfect" diet and exercise, she blows it. She doesn't understand why she does this to herself. She really does want to lose that 10 pounds, but she can never seem to stick to her diet long enough to pull it off. Why?

Plenty of people say they want to lose weight, but in reality, they do everything they can to sabotage themselves. Losing weight is as much about how you *think* as it is about what you *eat*. In order to truly be ready to be successful in weight loss, you need to be mentally ready. Take a moment to think about these questions:

ARE YOU WILLING TO MAKE LIFELONG LIFESTYLE CHANGES?

In order to be successful in taking off the weight, you have to be willing to make changes in your lifestyle that will last for good. Sitting on the couch, mindlessly munching on Cheetos must give way to standing in the kitchen to slice some apples for dessert.

Think about whether or not you're ready to make the changes you need to in order to reach your goal. Have you thought about the habits that you need to shake up? Roberta, forty-two, tried to lose weight dozens of times. It was only until after she realized she wasn't going on a diet, but instead needed to change her unwise eating habits, that the weight came off permanently.

HAVE YOU THOUGHT ABOUT WHAT'S WAYLAID YOUR EFFORTS IN THE PAST?

You haven't been able to lose the weight up until this point. Have you thought about why? Any major life events that might distract your efforts now? Marital problems, jobs stresses, financial worries?

Mary, thirty-four, hated her dead-end job at an insurance agency. She dreaded going into the office every day, and her only source of comfort was a big bar of chocolate. She'd try to resist, but every day at lunch and every night when she got home, eating that rich, creamy candy always took the edge off her miserable, stressful days.

After a particularly grueling week, Mary made a snap decision to quit her job. And immediately she felt lighter—mentally and physically. Suddenly, she no longer felt the urge for chocolate. She focused instead on scanning the papers and the Internet for a new job. By the time she found a new position, she'd lost five pounds.

Emotional eating is a big problem for many people. Anger, stress, boredom, or loneliness can trigger eating. Identify your triggers and make sure all your ducks are in order, so to speak, so you can seriously concentrate on your weight-loss program.

DO YOU HAVE A PARTNER YOU CAN DEPEND ON FOR EMOTIONAL HELP?

You're bound to face dozens of distractions, temptations, and reasons to become disheartened when you're driving down the road to permanent weight loss. Having someone to be accountable to can make things easier. It doesn't have to be a spouse or romantic partner. Buddy up with someone at work, or consider joining a weight-loss support group.

When Jamie turned forty, she decided that was the time to lose the 30 pounds she'd always wanted to get rid of. She called her best friend Lisa, and together the two went on the green coffee bean extract diet. They texted each other pictures of their scale weights every Friday, and called each other when they were tempted to eat a whole pint of ice cream. They also met four mornings a week at the gym, and used the time to gossip on the treadmill.

DO YOU HAVE A POSITIVE ATTITUDE ABOUT THE UPCOMING CHALLENGE?

Every time Liza, twenty-seven, would start a new diet she'd go into it with a sense of doom. She'd obsess over what she'd have to cut out of her life to get to the weight she wanted, and dreaded the thought of exercising every day. Monica, thirty-two, on the other hand, was excited about changing her eating habits. She'd felt sluggish and tired for years, and finally woke up one morning thinking, "There's got to be a way to feel better." Guess which woman lost the weight?

Are you excited about what lies ahead or do you shudder at the thought? If it's the latter, you're far more likely to jump ship the minute some rough water hits. Instead of being afraid of what's in front of you, try to welcome it. Think about how good you'll feel when you can fit into that little black dress or when someone compliments you on how great you look.

HOW MUCH DO YOU NEED TO LOSE?

Chances are, if you're reading this book, you want to lose some weight. Maybe you're having trouble zipping up your jeans. Or maybe you just don't like the way you look in the mirror. You might need to lose some weight in order to lower your risk of certain diseases. So how does your weight truly stack up objectively?

You may have heard the term body mass index but you're still not sure what it is. The BMI, for short, is a weight-to-height ratio that experts use to gauge body fat. To find out yours, use this calculation:

1. Multiply your height in inches by itself. For example, if you're five-foot-six, that's 66 inches. So multiply 66×66, which equals 4,356.
2. Now divide your weight in pounds by that number. So, if you weigh 158 pounds, you'd divide 158 by 4,356, which equals .03627.
3. Lastly, multiply that number by 704.5. This is your BMI, which here would be 25.5.

Or, you can use the table on page 32.
What number did you get?

- If your BMI is less than 18.5, you are considered underweight. Just as being overweight comes with health risks, being underweight comes with risks as well, so if your BMI falls within this range, speak to a doctor or nutritionist about what you can do to get your BMI up, so it's more within a normal range.
- If your BMI is 18.5 to 24.9, you are considered in the healthy weight range and should be commended. If you're more toward the higher end, you may still want to try the green coffee bean extract diet because you just don't *feel* you're the weight you want to be. Come on and join in. You won't believe how easy it is.
- If your BMI is 25.0 to 29.9, you are considered overweight. The good news: if you're on the lower end of the range, the increased risk to your health is modest and with just a few diet tweaks and the use of green coffee bean extract, you could easily get your weight down to the normal range. If your BMI is over 27, your health risks are beginning to rise significantly. The benefits of following our diet as well as taking green coffee bean extract is even more important for you.
- If your BMI is 30 to 35, you are considered obese. With

BODY MASS INDEX (BMI) TABLE

	NORMAL						OVERWEIGHT					OBESE										EXTREMELY OBESE														
BMI	19	20	21	22	23	24	25	26	27	28	29	30	31	32	33	34	35	36	37	38	39	40	41	42	43	44	45	46	47	48	49	50	51	52	53	54
Height (inches)																						Body Weight (pounds)														
58	91	96	100	105	110	115	119	124	129	134	138	143	148	153	158	162	167	172	177	181	186	191	196	201	205	210	215	220	224	229	234	239	244	248	253	258
59	94	99	104	109	114	119	124	128	133	138	143	148	153	158	163	168	173	178	183	188	193	198	203	208	212	217	222	227	232	237	242	247	252	257	262	267
60	97	102	107	112	118	123	128	133	138	143	148	153	158	163	168	174	179	184	189	194	199	204	209	215	220	225	230	235	240	245	250	255	261	266	271	276
61	100	106	111	116	122	127	132	137	143	148	153	158	164	169	174	180	185	190	195	201	206	211	217	222	227	232	238	243	248	254	259	264	269	275	280	285
62	104	109	115	120	126	131	136	142	147	153	158	164	169	175	180	186	191	196	202	207	213	218	224	229	235	240	246	251	256	262	267	273	278	284	289	295
63	107	113	118	124	130	135	141	146	152	158	163	169	175	180	186	191	197	203	208	214	220	225	231	237	242	248	254	259	265	270	278	282	287	293	299	304
64	110	116	122	128	134	140	145	151	157	163	169	174	180	186	192	197	204	209	215	221	227	232	238	244	250	256	262	267	273	279	285	291	296	302	308	314
65	114	120	126	132	138	144	150	156	162	168	174	180	186	192	198	204	210	216	222	228	234	240	246	252	258	264	270	276	282	288	294	300	306	312	318	324
66	118	124	130	136	142	148	155	161	167	173	179	186	192	198	204	210	216	223	229	235	241	247	253	260	266	272	278	284	291	297	303	309	315	322	328	334
67	121	127	134	140	146	153	159	166	172	178	185	191	198	204	211	217	223	230	236	242	249	255	261	268	274	280	287	293	299	306	312	319	325	331	338	344
68	125	131	138	144	151	158	164	171	177	184	190	197	203	210	216	223	230	236	243	249	256	262	269	276	282	289	295	302	308	315	322	328	335	341	348	354
69	128	135	142	149	155	162	169	176	182	189	196	203	209	216	223	230	236	243	250	257	263	270	277	284	291	297	304	311	318	324	331	338	345	351	358	365
70	132	139	146	153	160	167	174	181	188	195	202	209	216	222	229	236	243	250	257	264	271	278	285	292	299	306	313	320	327	334	341	348	355	362	369	376
71	136	143	150	157	165	172	179	186	193	200	208	215	222	229	236	243	250	257	265	272	279	286	293	301	308	315	322	329	338	343	351	358	365	372	379	387
72	140	147	154	162	169	177	184	191	199	206	213	221	228	235	242	250	258	265	272	279	287	294	302	309	316	324	331	338	346	353	361	368	375	383	390	397
73	144	151	159	166	174	182	189	197	204	212	219	227	235	242	250	257	265	272	280	288	295	302	310	318	325	333	340	348	355	363	371	378	386	393	401	408
74	148	155	163	171	179	186	194	202	210	218	225	233	241	249	256	264	272	280	287	295	303	311	319	326	334	342	350	358	365	373	381	389	396	404	412	420
75	152	160	168	176	184	192	200	208	216	224	232	240	248	256	264	272	279	287	295	303	311	319	327	335	343	351	359	367	375	383	391	399	407	415	423	431
76	156	164	172	180	189	197	205	213	221	230	238	246	254	263	271	279	287	295	304	312	320	328	336	344	353	361	369	377	385	394	402	410	418	426	435	443

Source: adopted from Clinical Guidelines on the Identification, Evaluation, and Treatment of Overweight and Obesity in Adults. The Evidence Report.

the risks to your health being higher, you will seriously benefit from the advice you will find in this book.

• If your BMI is over 35, you are severely obese and should see a health-care provider about losing weight.

BY THE NUMBERS

Everything today is rush, rush, rush. But when it comes to weight loss, slow and steady wins the race. Research shows that people who lose weight gradually and steadily—about one to two pounds per week—are more successful at keeping it off permanently. So while we're showing you a specific diet plan, it's really about an ongoing lifestyle that you can continue long after you've reached your weight-loss goal.

ESTIMATED CALORIE NEEDS PER DAY BY AGE, GENDER, AND PHYSICAL ACTIVITY LEVEL

This eating plan does not require you to measure foods or count calories. Still, it's probably a good idea for you to know approximately what you should be consuming, so you might want to take a look at the table below which gives you the estimated number of calories needed to maintain calorie balance for various gender and age groups at three different levels of physical activity. The estimates are rounded to the nearest 200 calories. Your own calorie needs may be higher or lower than these average estimates.

Now forget everything you've just read about BMIs and calorie needs. While it's good to have a yardstick on how much you should be eating, it's difficult, if not downright impossible, to calculate calories in the real world. So, take the calorie counting we've just taught you with the proverbial grain of salt. If you'd like to tally for a day or two to judge how much you're really eating, go ahead. But don't make yourself crazy. Remember, the

GENDER	AGE	SEDENTARY*	MODERATELY ACTIVE*	ACTIVE*
Females	19–30	1800–2000	2000–2200	2400
	31–50	1800	2000	2200
	51+	1600	1800	2000–2200
Males	19–30	2400–2600	2600-2800	3000
	31–50	2200–2400	2400-2600	2800-3000
	51+	2000–2200	2200-2400	2400-2800

*Sedentary means a lifestyle that includes only the light physical activity associated with typical day-to-day life.
*Moderately active means a lifestyle that includes physical activity equivalent to walking about 1.5 to 3 miles per day at 3 to 4 miles per hour, in addition to the light physical activity associated with typical day-to-day life.
*Active means a lifestyle that includes physical activity equivalent to walking more than 3 miles per day at 3 to 4 miles per hour, in addition to the light physical activity associated with typical day-to-day life.

green coffee bean extract study subjects lost weight even while sticking to their regular diets, so this doesn't have to be hard.

GET ON YOUR WAY

We know the green coffee bean extract diet works. But following the eating and exercise plan takes motivation. Lots of dieters do well for a time, but then, those Double Stuff Oreos come a calling, and, well, you know the rest. Good intentions can only last so long, so you need concrete techniques to help strengthen your resolve. Here are some stick-to-it strategies.

MOTIVATIONAL TIP #1: SET REALISTIC GOALS

Each time Karen, forty-five, started a diet she set her sights on losing 10 pounds in ten days. And every diet she went on lasted exactly ten days. When she failed to make her 10-pound goal, she gave up.

One of the strongest predictors for weight-loss success lies in what goals you've set out from the start. Losing 10 pounds in ten days is never going to happen, and you're just setting yourself up for failure. Instead of choosing an impossible goal, go with something sensible: you're going to drop one jean size (with no time limit), or you're going to the gym at least four times this week. Setting smaller benchmarks along the way will keep you motivated for the long haul.

MOTIVATIONAL TIP #2: LAY OUT YOUR END PRODUCT

It's great to have a picture in your mind of where you came from and where you want to go. Take that one step further and post your pictures. Snap a photo of yourself now and stick it on the refrigerator or on your bathroom mirror to remind yourself of where you once were. Then cut out a picture of someone whose figure you want to emulate (or find a picture of yourself at your thinnest if you've got one). Post that one around the house, too. Got a pair of skinny jeans you want to fit into? An itsy bitsy bikini? Hang something prominently in your closet and try it on every so often. Find something that you want more than the chocolate ice cream in your freezer and keep it where you can see it.

MOTIVATIONAL TIP #3: GO SLOWLY AND BE PATIENT

Changes don't happen overnight. You have a better chance at sticking with your plan, and keeping the weight off for the long term if you lose it slowly. If you're starving and deprived you'll be cranky and irritable and you're bound to throw in the towel early. Congratulate yourself on every small victory, whether it

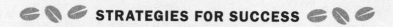 **STRATEGIES FOR SUCCESS**

Here are some tactics to insure a winning weight loss:

BUDDY UP: Studies have found that those who diet with a partner drop twice as many pounds than those who go it alone. Having someone who shares your concerns—and commitment—can make sticking with the diet easier.

RELIEVE STRESS, AND DON'T BE AFRAID TO ASK FOR HELP: When you're feeling life's pressures, it's tempting to grab a pint of Ben & Jerry's to help you feel better. Stop the pattern before it starts. Think back to some times in your life that have sent you running for the freezer. What would have happened if instead of eating you'd asked for whatever you were craving? For overall stress relief,

be a half pound on the scale or that you chose the stairs instead of the elevator.

MOTIVATIONAL TIP #4: SWEAT FOR SERVICE

Vicki, thirty-six, was overweight and out of shape and she realized she needed to make a change. But she had zero motivation to do anything. While thumbing through a magazine, she saw an ad for the Avon Walk for Breast Cancer. Although she'd never done any sort of race in her life, she thought it sounded like a rewarding thing to do. She got a group of coworkers to sign up with her, and with no way to turn back, she began a walking program to get ready.

Signing up for a charity walk or run is a great motivation to help you to get in shape. Not only will you feel good about helping a good cause, you'll feel so guilty after hitting up friends and family for donations, you'll have no choice but to try to finish first.

take up hobbies that can help you address stress in a way other than ice cream—take a yoga class, learn meditation, or try some tai chi.

WRITE IT DOWN: List everything you eat each day—and we mean everything (yes, that bite of your daughter's mac and cheese and the two handfuls of Nilla Wafers you ate count!). This will help you see in print what you've been eating, and will keep you accountable.

REWARD YOURSELF ALONG THE WAY: Celebrate the little victories, whether it's skipping your after-lunch chocolate bar or taking the stairs instead of the elevator. But, ahem, not with a hot fudge sundae! Take a bubble bath, get a mani/pedi, or treat yourself to a new pair of strappy sandals.

Quiz: What's Keeping You Fat?

There are dozens of different reasons why people gain weight. And even more reasons why they can't take the weight off. Take the quiz below to see what's led you down this path, and get some hints on what road to take to get to thin.

Which of the following questions most accurately describes you at the end of the day?

a. I just feel like plopping down on the coach. Alone. I'm depressed and could use a cookie for a boost.

b. I'm totally overwhelmed. There's never enough time in the day to do everything I need to do.

c. I'm ravenous. I haven't eaten anything all day and need to make up for it now by eating everything in sight

Which of the following statements do you agree with most strongly?

    a. I regularly worry about my finances, getting sick, or disappointing my friends and family.

    b. I'd love to take a healthy-cooking class, but who the heck has time?

    c. Everyone in my family has always struggled with their weight. My genes make it impossible for me to ever fit into skinny jeans.

When I see a slice of chocolate cake . . .

    a. I close my eyes and dig in.

    b. I put it aside to eat at the end of the day.

    c. I try my best to avoid it altogether. But in the end, I usually eat the slice. And another. And, often the entire cake.

When I've gone on diets before . . .

    a. I do okay for a while. Then I get into a fight with my husband, or my kids don't listen to me, and diet goes down the drain.

    b. I find it impossible to find the time cook healthy foods for myself and exercise. Who has the strength?

    c. I've lost the weight really quickly, but it inevitably comes back twice as fast.

On a typical weeknight, my dinner usually consists of . . .

    a. Whatever I'm in the mood for. Maybe pizza, maybe Chinese, or maybe even mac and cheese if I've had a really bad day.

    b. Whatever's on my kids' plates, or I eat fast food in the car while shuttling everyone around.

    c. Depends. If I'm on a diet? A frozen diet meal. If I'm not dieting, anything I want.

On weekends I . . .

    a. Eat way too much. I rarely feel satisfied and feel the urge to snack throughout the day.

    b. Am never sitting down. Between Girl Scouts and soccer practice, there's no time for a real meal.

    c. Don't eat all day. I have to save my calories so I can binge at those dinners out.

Mostly As: You're super emotional and probably eat more than you should for comfort. Take a look at who's around you. Do you have an emotional support system? If not, consider joining a Mommy and Me group or find a community outreach program. Volunteering at a local soup kitchen would be a good outlet for you as well. Seeing those less fortunate will make you realize that your life isn't as bad as you think it is.

Mostly Bs: Your lifestyle is hindering your weight loss. You need to reach out more to family and friends for help. You also need to prep and plan ahead so you don't have to make last-minute food decisions while you're starving. With just a little forethought, you could be at your goal weight in no time.

Mostly Cs: Your eating habits and lack of nutrition knowledge are what's been holding you back. You've probably also yo-yo dieted for years, which has sent your metabolism on a roller coaster. Read this book carefully. We'll probably dispel a lot of what you thought you knew.

CHAPTER 5

Stories of Success

By now you're probably ready to get started on our amazing new eating plan . . . but we want to excite you even more. So before you begin, take a few minutes to read about the women in this chapter who have succeeded in shedding pounds with the help of the green coffee bean extract diet. Chances are, whether you want to lose 5 pounds or 55, you'll get inspiration from the women who have followed our eating and exercise plan . . . and won the war against the weight.

NORMA, FORTY-ONE

Norma was one of those lucky girls growing up: she could pack in truckloads of food and never seem to gain an ounce. The blonde-haired beauty stood at five foot eight and 124 pounds. When everyone was gaining the freshman 15 in college, Norma held her weight steady. On the first day of her sophomore year she met Larry, who asked her to marry him on the day they graduated. Larry immediately got a job at a New York City brokerage firm, and the two set up house in a tony suburb.

Although Norma lunched often with girlfriends and ate whatever she wanted, she played tennis at the club three to four times a week, and her weight never fluctuated. Until she got pregnant with twins, and had to go on bedrest at twenty-one weeks. "I could only get out of bed to bathe and go to the bathroom," she says, and her metabolism slowed to near nothing.

After she delivered twin girls, she figured she'd get back to her pre pregnancy weight, but caring for two babies left little time to plan meals, and tennis at the club was out of the question. Although Larry urged her to get a babysitter so she'd have time for herself, Norma said she'd waited too long for her girls to hand them off to a nanny.

By the time her girls were five she'd ballooned up to 180 pounds. Although the girls loved to run around in the park, Norma would huff and puff to keep up with them. And sitting on the floor to play board games was near impossible. Although most of the time she refused to let anyone take pictures of her, on the twins' sixth birthday, her mother-in-law convinced her to be in a family shot, and when she saw the picture a few weeks later, she was mortified. "I couldn't believe how heavy I'd gotten!" she says. She vowed to do something that very day.

Norma had read about green coffee bean extract and thought it couldn't hurt to try. After getting the okay from her doctor, she picked up a package of the capsules at the drug store and took a look at her pantry. "When I really looked at it I couldn't believe how many unhealthy foods were in there!" she says. "I had always used the excuse that the junk I bought were for the girls, but how is that an excuse? Why should I be feeding my family such unhealthy stuff?"

She threw out all the processed junk, though she knew she couldn't completely give up all her food vices. Ice cream had always been Norma's weakness, and she wanted to be able to enjoy it once in a while. Norma decided to take it one step at a time, her first step being to cut all the processed food she'd been eating. Her first week she dropped 2.5 pounds.

Next, she tried to tackle her paltry intake of vegetables and fruit. Potatoes were the only vegetable she'd eaten for years, but a trip to the food store yielded eggplant, zucchini, sweet potatoes, and peppers, plus apples, bananas, and watermelon. Her goal was to eat at least one to two servings of fruit or vegetables at each meal, and she found that if she did that, she wasn't all that hungry for junk. If she did need something sweet, she reached for watermelon or strawberries first, and she found that usually satisfied her craving. And, of course, she took her green coffee bean extract before every meal.

Within a month Norma had dropped eight pounds. She was thrilled! She decided to add some exercise into the mix to see if she could get the weight to come off faster. She still felt too self-conscious to try tennis again, so she used her time with the girls at the park to exercise. Instead of sitting on the bench like she usually did, Norma stood and walked around as the girls playing on the monkey bars. And when the girls asked her to push them on the swing, instead of saying no, she swung them high in the air.

Before she knew it, Norma had lost 40 pounds. She felt better and more energetic than she'd felt since before she had the children. She also felt sharper and smarter than she had in a long time. "I'm not sure if it's from the green coffee bean extract or because I can just sleep better at night, but I don't care. Whatever it is, I'll take it!" she says. And tennis? She's playing again—four times a week.

VALERIE, FIFTY-EIGHT

At only five feet, Valerie had to watch what she ate her entire life. "You can see every ounce on me, so I need to be super super careful," she says. For the majority of the time, Valerie stuck to complex carbs, lean meats and fish, low-fat dairy, and plenty of vegetables and fruit. Her treats were limited to no-fat frozen yogurt and the occasional square of dark chocolate for its antioxidants.

Although she suffered from a bit of arthritis in her knees, Valerie still managed to get to the gym at least four to five mornings a week before she headed to her job as a real estate agent.

And even when she missed a workout, showing houses all day made for a workout in itself. "I wouldn't say it was easy, but being careful helped me keep my weight to where I wanted it to be. Plus I just felt better eating healthfully and moving my body as much as possible."

When she hit menopause, things began to change. Valerie felt the weight creeping up a bit and although she tried to cut down on portion size, to keep her weight constant she ended up cutting her diet so much she was down to eating only lettuce leaves all day. But still, Valerie's jeans got more and more snug. When she couldn't zipper her favorite pair of skinny jeans, she knew it was time to do something different.

Someone at her office had lost weight with green coffee bean extract and she thought she'd like to try it. She started taking the capsules and a miraculous thing happened. Even though she had added some foods into her diet (she knew she couldn't subsist on lettuce leaves forever), she lost a pound that first week. She realized that she'd cut so many calories out of her diet that her body had gone into starvation mode, burning the few calories she did take in more efficiently. So adding food back in, coupled with the green coffee bean extract actually helped the weight come off. Within six weeks she was back in her skinny jeans. "I couldn't believe that adding food *into* my diet could actually help me lose weight!"

SUZY, TWENTY-FOUR

Suzy was chubby as a kid, but when Suzy turned fourteen, her sister was killed in a car accident, and Suzy's weight ballooned. By the time she reached college she was 60 pounds overweight. After graduating she decided she had to do something. "I hadn't been invited to my prom, I'd never been on a school sport, and I'd never even had a boyfriend. I realized I was missing out on so much in life because of my weight."

Some friends at school had been talking about this great new diet they'd tried, so she decided to give it a go and after speaking to her doctor, Suzy bought a month's supply of green coffee bean extract. She focused on making one change at a time, setting her sights first on her love of simple carbs. So she vowed to not eat anything white—no pasta, no mashed potatoes, no sugar cookies. Within a few weeks she was down 10 pounds.

Then she looked for another goal: She'd exercise fifteen to twenty minutes a day, three to four times a week. She did that, and the weight came off even faster. She then cut out all fried food from her diet, then switched from the high-fatty meats she loved to lean chicken, beef, and especially fish. "The only fish I'd ever had before was the Fish Fillet at McDonald's, but when I tried salmon grilled with a little lemon, I realized I really liked it." Soon she was not only exercising fifteen to twenty minutes a day, she was turning her back on the bus and walking to work instead. "Not only did I get an extra thirty minutes of activity in, I also saved a bundle of money!"

Suzy still had a few vices—she loved her daily dose of chocolate, which she allowed herself to indulge in at the end of every workout. If she didn't get to the gym, she skipped the chocolate treat. "It was a great motivator," she says.

Before she knew it, Suzy was fitting into a size six pair of jeans—something she never thought she'd do. Her friends wanted to set her up on dates right and left, and within a few months of getting to her goal weight she met the love of her life—on a bike trail! "The green coffee bean extract diet saved my life—in more ways than one!" she says.

VICKI, TWENTY-SIX

Vicki wanted to lose weight for her June wedding. "I wasn't overweight, but I wanted to trim down a bit so when I walked down the aisle in my mermaid-style dress, everyone would say

'Wow!'" Vicki had heard about a great new supplement and diet plan, so she picked up a copy of the book and got started right away. "I didn't want to follow a meal plan that was laid out for me, so I decided to try a few of the tricks in the book," she says.

Vicki has always skipped breakfast—she never had time to eat—so she prepped the ingredients for a smoothie at night, and stored the blender in the fridge. "It only took me a minute to blend up a delicious breakfast, and just doing that helped me not become ravenous at 11:00 A.M. every day," she says. Vicki also made sure to eat at least five servings of vegetables a day, and she switched from white grains to whole grains. "Even though I should have been exhausted planning my wedding, I actually had more energy than I had before!"

With just those small tweaks, and the help of the green coffee bean extract, Vicki lost five pounds in a month. At her final fitting, the seamstress had to take in her wedding dress. "I couldn't believe how easy it was." And on the day of her wedding, everyone was completely wowed. Mission accomplished.

MELANIE, THIRTY-TWO

Melanie, a dark-haired beauty, had never had a problem with her weight. It would fluctuate up and down five or so pounds depending on the season, but on her five-foot-seven body, nobody really noticed. But when Melanie's life began to spin out of control, so did her weight.

"The publishing company I'd worked at for four years cut back, so I got laid off. And I found out my boyfriend was cheating on me!" The only comfort Melanie had was in a bowl of macaroni and cheese. Or a bowl of ice cream. "I never looked in the mirror during that time. I just spent the day sitting, looking at the newspaper or surfing the Internet, searching for a job, with a big bowl of potato chips beside me."

Quite quickly her weight ballooned to 168 pounds. When her

severance pay ran out after six months, Melanie realized she better do something. And fast. "I knew I had to start going out and interviewing for jobs, so I looked in the closet to see if any of my work clothes would still fit me. Wow, did it hit me. The clothes weren't tight—they were completely unwearable. I'd been in total denial about how heavy I'd gotten."

Melanie had never dieted in her life, so she went to the library to check out some diet books. Most of the plans just didn't thrill her. "They were all full of rules about how you can't eat carbs or you can't eat more than 1200 calories a day or you can't eat any sugar or flour. Who needs that?" But one diet did suit her—the green coffee bean extract diet. "I liked the fact that you could eat anything you wanted, within reason, of course," Melanie says. She began taking the supplement and following the meal program laid out in the book. And she realized that dieting was easier than she thought.

She still sat down with a bowl—but this time she favored bowls of broth-based soups. She found if she ate soup before a meal she could rarely even finish all the food she'd put on her plate. She also began to walk every morning, before she'd start on her job search.

Melanie spoke with dozens of potential employers over the phone, and when she finally got called—by her former company's largest competitor—she was excited. But also nervous as she stepped into her closet to see if she had anything to wear. As she put one leg into her favorite black pants she held her breath . . . and they fit! Melanie looked in the mirror after she was all dressed and was elated to see her old body back again. Feeling confident, she aced the interview and landed the job.

JUDI, TWENTY-NINE

Judi was an athlete her entire life. She played volleyball, soccer, and ran track in high school, and throughout college she played on a recreational softball league. When she landed a job as an insurance broker, she was excited to find that the company had a softball team and she joined immediately.

One evening during practice, as Judi was rounding the bases, her foot buckled under and she fell to the ground. A coworker took her to the emergency room and she'd severely broken two bones in her foot. In a cast for three months, Judi couldn't do a thing. Except eat her mother's delicious pasta. Her mother loaded Judi's plate with pasta, meatballs, and sausage, and Judi lost herself in the food. By the time the cast came off she was 15 pounds heavier.

Judi had heard about the green coffee bean diet, and began the meal plans right away. "I love to cook, so preparing the recipes laid out in the book was enjoyable, and the foods were delicious." That's not to say she didn't enjoy the occasional indulgence. "Every Sunday I'd visit my mom and I'd eat everything she served me. Pasta Alfredo, sausage, and peppers. You name it, I'd eat it." But Monday morning she'd go right back on the green coffee bean extract diet meal plan.

After finishing a round of physical therapy, Judi was able to resume her normal sports routine, which helped the weight come off faster. She couldn't believe how easy it all was. "People always say that dieting is hard, but really, the green coffee bean extract diet was a cinch!"

Judi got to her goal weight the day her softball team reached the world series. "I was in total fighting form," she brags. And fight she did. Her team won the game, 5–2. Judi felt like a champion in more ways than one.

CHAPTER 6

Tempting Meal Plans to Get You Started . . . And Keep You Satisfied

Now you've learned all about the groundbreaking supplement that has folks all over the country talking, and you've seen the research. You've also learned about dietary supplements and what you should look for when shopping for one that is safe and delivers what the label promises. Now it's time to start eating, enjoying, and losing pounds.

In this chapter we're going to lay out the revolutionary new meal plan that will help get you to the weight you want to be without feeling hungry or watching every morsel you put in your mouth. Keep in mind, even if you do fall victim to a chocolate chip cookie or two, as long as you keep taking your green coffee bean extract, you should continue to lose weight. If you want to supercharge your weight loss, follow the plan we've mapped out for you, and you'll get to your goal that much faster, feeling satisfied and loving the way you look.

PUMP UP THE VOLUME

So many diets fail because they're based on deprivation—you can't eat this and you can't eat that. What's so great about the green coffee bean extract diet is that you can eat a lot of delicious, health-supporting foods that don't pack on the pounds. So you'll never be hungry and you'll never feel like you're lacking anything. We mean it. You can eat more food, feel fuller, and actually be reducing your total caloric intake. At the same time, you'll train your body to expect and enjoy foods that are good for you, so you'll stop craving those processed, empty-calorie foods.

The key is to choose the right foods. Instead of picking measly portions of low-volume foods, you can eat large portions of high-volume foods that have fewer calories per bite, filling you up on a smaller number of calories. So you get a lot of fullness bang for your calorie buck. We're not talking about ho-hum rice cakes and celery stalks. We mean foods that pack a lot of flavor and satisfy your need for texture and variety.

What we're talking about is a concept known as calorie density. Think back to your high school science classes. Remember what density means? It's the distribution of a quantity per unit. In this case, the *distribution of quantity* is calories and the *unit* is the particular amount of food.

High-calorie-dense foods have a great deal of calories packed in a small amount of food. Think cheddar cheese (or most full-fat cheeses). A single ounce of cheddar is only one inch square, but it packs 100 calories into that one little cube. Low-calorie density means there are not a lot of calories spread out over a whole lot of food. Take romaine lettuce, which is packed with vitamins A and C. You would have to eat *more than 10 cups of shredded romaine* to consume the same 100 calories you find in one tiny cube of cheese. Obviously, when you're watching your weight, you want to eat a lot of high-volume, low-calorie-dense foods, so you'll be able to eat a greater amount of food that will leave you feeling more satisfied, while still consuming fewer calories.

WHAT MAKES A FOOD LOW IN CALORIE DENSITY?

The three most important factors that contribute to the calorie density of food are:

- **WATER.** The more water you find in a food, the lower the calorie density. Why? Because water has zero calories, but it takes up a lot of weight and space. So, foods that are higher in water—like a grapefruit, for example—take up a lot of space, but half a grapefruit is only 39 calories.
- **FIBER.** Foods that are higher in fiber tend to be less in calorie density as well. And high-fiber foods bring with them another benefit: they take longer to digest, making you feel full longer on fewer calories.
- **FAT.** At the opposite end of the calorie-density spectrum, fat is the most calorie dense component of food, providing more than twice as many calories per gram as carbohydrates or protein. One teaspoon of butter, for example, contains almost the same number of calories as two whole cups of raw broccoli.

To figure out the calorie density of a food, divide the calories by the number of grams in a serving (listed on the nutrition label). For example, a food that has 100 calories and weighs 200 grams (about 7 ounces) has a calorie density of 0.5. For the most part, a low-calorie-dense food is one that's below 1.0. But we don't want you to get too bogged down by the numbers. We'll show you how simple it really can be later in this chapter.

RULES TO EAT BY

Very soon, we'll give you a suggested meal plan, but that doesn't mean you have to follow it to the letter. In fact, you don't have to follow it at all. If you're taking the green coffee bean extract, you're bound to lose weight no matter how you eat. However, if you want to supersize your weight loss (and who doesn't want to supersize their weight loss?), you can follow our list of suggested menus (starting on page 56), or you can follow your own healthy eating plan, and just incorporate the following suggestions.

DON'T GO HUNGRY.

Our meal plans provide three meals and two snacks per day. Whether you follow our meal plan or create your own, always make sure to eat enough healthy, high-volume, low-calorie foods to avoid hunger. Remember, you don't have to starve yourself to lose weight with your green coffee bean extract. In fact, if you feel your stomach rumbling, that means you're not eating enough.

However, make sure that when you're hungry, it's truly the physical kind. Before you reach to open the fridge, ask yourself, "What am I hungry for?" If you're mad, sad, or bored, it's not food that's calling. See if something else—a call to a friend, a walk in the fresh air, or a chapter of your favorite novel—will make the feeling go away.

And remember that there's a difference between a snack and a treat. A snack is a small amount of food to satisfy your hunger in between meals. A treat is something a bit more indulgent—a small scoop of frozen yogurt, a few cookies, a piece of dark chocolate—that you might enjoy once in a while.

CHOOSE YOUR CARBS WISELY.

Steer clear of anything made with refined white flour, which is converted into sugars very quickly, causing spikes and drops in blood sugar, and will probably send you running to the nearest vending machine. High-fiber foods, on the other hand, as we've mentioned, are low in calorie density, so you can eat more of them for fewer calories.

They also move more slowly through your digestive tract, helping you feel fuller longer. Swap white bread for whole wheat, sub in whole-wheat pasta for plain, and choose brown rice over white whenever possible. There are other interesting grains such as quinoa, farro, and barley. High in fiber and protein, these grains offer a nutty texture and an alternative to the same old, same old.

ALWAYS LEAVE THE TABLE SATISFIED.

If you feel a meal isn't doing it for you, feel free to add anything from the list of foods (page 60) to bulk it up. The fuller you feel, the less likely you are to throw in the towel. Remember, though, feeling satisfied isn't the same as feeling so full you can't eat another bite. One of the lessons you should learn while you're on this diet is that *because* you can eat whatever you want, you won't always feel the need to stuff yourself silly.

BANISH THE WORD "CHEAT" FROM YOUR VOCABULARY.

We already said you should eat when you're hungry. Take that one step further and give yourself permission to treat yourself to the occasional goody. When we deprive ourselves of our favorite foods, we end up feeling guilty if we indulge in them. And then we feel like we've done something wrong, which usually sends us diving head-first into the cookie bin.

On this diet, dipping into the cookie bin is okay now and then— you've got your green coffee extract to help you lose the weight regardless. Yes, this diet gives you permission to eat those foods that are forbidden on most diets. Once you allow yourself to eat those two cookies, you'll no longer feel the need to eat the whole box. When you stop focusing on eating less, you'll actually start to eat less. And you'll stop wanting those foods that seemed so forbidden before. So, remember, a dip in the cookie bin every once in a while isn't going to kill your entire diet. Just don't make a habit of it if you want to lose weight steadily.

CHOOSE FOODS WITH MORE AIR AND MORE WATER.

This tricks your senses into thinking you've eaten more than you actually have. Think apples over apple juice, gelatin over

☕ ◖ ☕ SOUP UP YOUR WEIGHT LOSS ☕ ◖ ☕

A great low-calorie-dense food is broth-based soup. In fact, research done at Penn State University showed that when participants ate a first course of soup before a lunch entrée, they reduced their total calorie intake at lunch by 20 percent, compared to when they did not eat soup. Another study found that when people ate a broth-based soup before lunch they ate less than if they were given the same number of calories in an appetizer of cheese and crackers. The large helping of soup is more satisfying, and more filling, than the high-calorie-dense cheese and crackers. Eating soup as a first course also helps slow down your eating speed, so it can naturally give your brain a chance to catch up to your stomach.

ice cream, air-popped popcorn instead of pretzel nuggets. Three cups of salad with a light or low-fat dressing instead of a sandwich stuffed with meat and cheese. Fluffy foods and foods with irregular shapes will also make you think you're eating more.

LIMIT SATURATED FATS, AND USE GOOD FATS WISELY.

Good fats, like fatty fish, can be eaten in abundance. Evidence is mounting that omega-3 fatty acids are extremely beneficial for your health, including helping to reduce inflammation, helping to reduce the risk of chronic diseases such as heart disease, cancer, and arthritis. Omega-3 fatty acids also appear to be vital for cognitive behavior.

The American Heart Association recommends eating fish

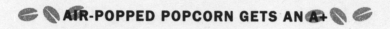

AIR-POPPED POPCORN GETS AN A+

This good-for-you nosh is surprisingly low in calories for the amount you get—just 30 calories per cup (without butter). And because of the irregular shape, popcorn fluffs up to looking like a lot of food! Keep it on hand for a Friday-night movie at home. For savory snacks, try this: lightly mist popcorn with olive oil and sprinkle with grated Parmesan cheese and cracked pepper, or cover with grated lime zest and chili powder. Craving something sweet? Throw some dark chocolate shavings in the bowl, or sprinkle with butter spray and a bit of brown sugar.

(particularly fatty fish like salmon, mackerel, herring, and lake trout) at least two times per week. Other fats, such as the fats you find in olives, olive oil, avocados, and nuts, are also good for you.

THREE WEEKS OF DAILY MENUS

The following menus are chockful of low-calorie, high-volume foods that are loaded with nutrition. And have we mentioned delicious? Foods you never thought you could eat on a diet, like frozen yogurt, tropical fruit salads, falafel, pancakes, and even pastas.

But here's the really exciting part—you don't have to follow these meal plans to the letter. In fact, you don't have to follow them at all. They're just suggestions. You've got the green coffee bean extract as a helpmate. So you can mix and match menus, or you can sub in your own meal every once in a while. Or you can skip the meal plans altogether and just create your own high-volume menu.

THE "WHOLE" TRUTH

When looking at a package label, make sure you're truly getting whole grain. "Enriched flour," "degerminated," "unbleached wheat flour," and "wheat flour" are not whole grains. Even products labeled "whole grain" or "whole wheat" are often made with white flour as the main ingredient. Look for products that specify "100 percent whole grain" or "100 percent whole wheat" before plunking down cash for a product.

And if you're craving pepperoni pizza, go ahead and enjoy it guilt-free. Going out with friends on a Saturday night? Have that margarita (or two). Don't feel like you're doing anything wrong. Don't do it every other night, of course, but as long as you're incorporating most of the rules above, and taking your green coffee bean extract, the once-in-a-while delight won't destroy your weight-loss efforts.

Later in the chapter we'll also give you a list of free foods foods you can add into your diet so that you'll never feel famished. And we have some suggestions on how to make these foods even more delicious. The menus also feature some scrumptious recipes so you can tempt your taste buds with foods that are not only yummy, but optimal for your health as well. Remember, your goal is to lose weight while enjoying what you eat, when you eat it, without denying yourself anything.

As for drinks, try to stick to water or flavored seltzers as much as possible. Or try adding a splash or two of your favorite juice to seltzer and you'll be surprised at how much the resulting beverage will taste like a delicious light soda.

Coffee and tea are okay, too, though don't go overboard with the sugar substitutes. (See chapter 10 for more on sugar substitutes.)

Unlike other weight-loss plans, we don't think you should weigh and measure your food. Again, that just smacks of the I'm-on-a-diet deprivation that we want you to avoid. Instead, we want you to understand that some foods should take up a lot of space on your plate and others, not so much. So when you're planning your menus, keep your protein amounts to the size of your fist (or a deck of cards) and pile on the veggies. Grains should take up about a quarter of the space on your plate. If you're not sure how much to serve yourself, assume one serving (look on package labels for each food to gauge how much to give yourself). And remember to take your green coffee bean extract thirty minutes before each meal.

WEEK ONE

Monday

Green coffee bean extract capsules, taken as directed thirty minutes before each meal

Breakfast
Strawberry-Orange Breakfast Smoothie (page 74)

Lunch
White Bean and Broccoli Salad (page 79)
Whole-grain roll
Plum

Dinner
Linguine with Shrimp (page 87)
Salad with carrots, multi-colored peppers, onions, tomatoes, and cabbage with Dijon vinaigrette dressing
Oranges with Strawberry Sauce (page 95)

Two snacks (to have between meals if you feel hungry)
Nonfat yogurt with raspberries
Oatmeal with honey and low-fat milk

Tuesday

Green coffee bean extract capsules, taken as directed thirty minutes before each meal

Breakfast
Tropical Fruit Salad with mango (page 79)
Whole-Grain Buttermilk Pancakes with maple syrup (page 75)

Lunch
Pasta, Broccoli, and Basil Salad (page 80)

Dinner
Tilapia in Spicy Tomato Sauce (page 88)
Baked Sweet Potato Fries (page 100)
Steamed kale drizzled with olive oil and ginger
Almond Angel Food Cake with Mango Puree (page 96)

Two snacks (to have between meals if you feel hungry)
Whole-Wheat Garlic Chips (page 101)
Low-fat cottage cheese with grapes

Wednesday

Green coffee bean extract capsules, taken as directed thirty minutes before each meal

Breakfast
Bran flakes with blueberries and milk
Orange

Lunch
Turkey or ham sandwich on wheat roll
Lettuce, tomato, cucumber, onions
Fruit sorbet

Dinner
Baked pork chop rubbed with plenty of spices (see page 73 for
    ideas)
Wild rice
Steamed asparagus and broccoli with a lemon squeeze

Two snacks (to have between meals if you feel hungry)
Watermelon
Slice of low-fat cheese

Thursday

Green coffee bean extract capsules, taken as directed thirty
minutes before each meal

Breakfast
Whole-Grain Buttermilk Pancakes (page 75)
Blueberries

Lunch
Falafel with pita, lettuce, and tomato with cumin-spiced yogurt
    sauce (page 89)

Dinner
Chicken Chili (page 90)
Oat Groats with Carrots and Parsley (page 102)
Strawberries in Balsamic Vinegar (page 97)

Two snacks (to have between meals if you feel hungry)
Buttermilk with dried figs
Two Oatmeal Cookies (page 97)

Friday

Green coffee bean extract capsules, taken as directed thirty minutes before each meal

Breakfast
Broiled Grapefruit (page 75)
Fruit and Nut Granola with low-fat milk (page 76)

Lunch
Sweet Potato–Orange Soup (page 80)
Oriental Chicken and Bean Salad (page 81)

Dinner
Chicken Burgers served over chopped greens and tomatoes
    (page 91)
Steamed broccoli with spices
Brown Rice (page 103)
Papaya Sorbet (page 98)

Two snacks (to have between meals if you feel hungry)
Four sesame crackers with low-fat milk
Carrots with hummus

Saturday

Green coffee bean extract capsules, taken as directed thirty minutes before each meal

Breakfast
Bran flakes with strawberries and low-fat milk

Lunch
Split Pea Soup (page 82)
Shrimp and Black Bean Salad (page 82)

NEVER FEEL LIKE YOU'RE HUNGRY!

On this diet you should never hear your tummy growling. At any time of day or night, feel free to eat unlimited portions of the low-calorie-dense foods listed below. And if shredded carrots or other plain veggies don't appeal to you, we promise, you'll find that they tempt your taste buds if you toss them with the exciting sauces and toppings that we suggest in the box (on page 66).

- Artichokes
- Arugula
- Asparagus
- Bell peppers
- Berries
- Broccoli
- Broccoli sprouts
- Broth-based soups (chicken, onion, minestrone, vegetable, miso, etc.)
- Brussels sprouts
- Cabbage
- Cantaloupe
- Carrots
- Cauliflower
- Celery
- Chard
- Collard greens
- Dandelion greens
- Eggplant
- Gelatin desserts
- (high sugar) Honeydew
- Jalapenos
- Kale
- Lettuce
- Mushrooms
- Mustard greens
- Onions
- Peas
- Radishes
- Strawberries
- Spinach
- String beans
- Tofu
- Tomato
- Watermelon
- Non- or low-fat yogurt, unsweetened
- Zucchini

Dinner
Green salad (try a new veggie on it today—how about radishes?),
    with fat-free dressing of your choice
Grilled Salmon with Spinach and White Beans (page 91)
Carrots with Cumin (page 103)
Frozen Banana Dessert (page 99)

Two snacks (to have between meals if you feel hungry)
Pear
Strawberry Yogurt and Fruit (page 105)

Sunday

Green coffee bean extract capsules, taken as directed thirty
minutes before each meal

Breakfast
Orange
Oat Bran Bread French Toast with Glazed Apples (page 77)

Lunch
Tuna and Black-Eyed Pea Salad (page 83)

Dinner
Pork Medallions with Black Beans (page 92)
Brussels Sprouts with Shallots (page 104)
Ginger Baked Apple (page 100)

Two snacks (to have between meals if you feel hungry)
Bran flakes with low-fat milk
Vegetable Lentil Soup (page 84)

WEEK 2

Monday

Green coffee bean extract capsules, taken as directed thirty minutes before each meal

Breakfast
Whole-wheat English muffin
Slice Swiss cheese
Grapefruit

Lunch
Sliced Steak and Roasted Tomato Salad (page 85)
Diced strawberries with kiwi

Dinner
Shepherd's Pie with Sweet Potato Topping (page 93)
Summer Tomato Salad (page 85)
Cantaloupe Granita (page 99)

Two snacks (to have between meals if you feel hungry)
Tropical Citrus Shake (page 106)
Whole-wheat roll with peanut butter

Tuesday

Green coffee bean extract capsules, taken as directed thirty minutes before each meal

Breakfast
Low-fat Greek yogurt
Blueberries

Lunch
Spinach salad made with multicolored peppers, red onions, tomatoes, rinsed black beans, sliced avocado, and extra-virgin olive oil and apple cider vinegar dressing

Dinner
Grilled salmon sprinkled with ginger
Braised Red Cabbage (page 103)
Roasted cauliflower and Brussels sprouts
Sweet potato

Two snacks (to have between meals if you feel hungry)
Handful of walnuts
Cherries

Wednesday

Green coffee bean extract capsules, taken as directed thirty minutes before each meal

Breakfast
Two low-fat waffles
Blueberries

Lunch
Tomato soup
Part-skim mozzarella cheese on slice of whole-wheat toast
Big salad of romaine, tomato, onion, green and red peppers
Pear

Dinner
Chicken breast grilled, broiled, or baked
Brown rice
Steamed string beans with lemon ginger dressing

Two snacks (to have between meals if you feel hungry)
Whole-wheat dinner roll with almond butter
Low-fat yogurt

Thursday

Green coffee bean extract capsules, taken as directed thirty minutes before each meal

Breakfast
Potato-Kale Frittata (page 77)
Mixed fresh fruit cocktail
Slice whole-wheat toast

Lunch
Chicken–Wild Rice Salad with Mango and Ginger (page 86)

Dinner
Tomato-stuffed Pork Tenderloin with Roasted Poblano Sauce
   (page 94)
Roasted butternut squash with sprinkle of cinnamon
Steamed fresh spinach

Two snacks (to have between meals if you feel hungry)
Parsley–White Bean Dip with carrots, celery, green peppers, and
   red peppers (page 104)
Air-popped popcorn

Friday

Green coffee bean extract capsules, taken as directed thirty minutes before each meal

Breakfast
Oatmeal with cinnamon

Lunch
Vegetable Lentil Soup (page 84)
Tuna and Black-Eyed Pea Salad (page 83)

Dinner
Tilapia in Spicy Tomato Sauce (page 88)
Baked Sweet Potato Fries (page 100)
Steamed kale

Two snacks (to have between meals if you feel hungry)
Almond Angel Food Cake with Mango Puree (page 96)
Half grapefruit

Saturday

Green coffee bean extract capsules, taken as directed thirty minutes before each meal

Breakfast
Broiled Grapefruit (page 75)
Whole-wheat English muffin with two slices of low-fat cheese

Lunch
Ham sandwich on 6-inch wheat roll
Slice cheese
Lettuce, tomato, cucumber, onions
Half-cup fruit sorbet

Dinner
Ginger-soy marinated London Broil with roasted tomatoes
Roasted butternut squash with sprinkle of cinnamon
Steamed fresh spinach sprinkled with lemon and olive oil

Two snacks (to have between meals if you feel hungry)
Fennel and Orange Salad with Parsley and Olives (page 87)
Oatmeal with cinnamon

GET SAUCY!

While the idea of celery stalks may not send your heart racing, be-dazzling with condiments and dressings can make any snack sing. Try dressing up your free foods with some of the following. And for a more indulgent feel without many extra calories, add a few drops of olive or sesame oil.

- Vinegar
- Lemon juice
- Salsa
- Curry paste (comes in jars)
- Non-fat mayonnaise
- Fat-free dressings (forget old-school Italian dressing— try sesame or miso)

- Soy sauce
- Worcestershire sauce
- Barbecue sauce
- Horseradish
- Ketchup
- Mustard
- Relish

Or, invent your own accoutrements. Create a dipping sauce with soy, lemon juice and ginger, chop some mango into salsa for a sweet twist on a Mexican favorite, or throw together some apple cider vinegar, pomegranate juice, extra-virgin olive oil, and honey for a tangy dressing. A few drops of sesame oil will give any dipping sauce an Asian flair. If you like garlic, go for it. It's great added to dipping sauces and vinaigrettes. Add Tabasco or another hot sauce of your liking to make your food spicy. Play around to keep things exciting!

Sunday

Green coffee bean extract capsules, taken as directed thirty minutes before each meal

Breakfast
Fresh sliced cantaloupe
Pumpkin-Nut Quick Bread (page 78)

Lunch
Lean turkey sandwich on whole-grain roll with lettuce, spinach,
    onions, and tomatoes
Minestrone soup

Dinner
Grilled salmon drizzled with olive oil and parsley
Medium sweet potato
Steamed broccoli and carrots

Two snacks (to have between meals if you feel hungry)
Low-fat yogurt
Whole-wheat English muffin with almond butter

WEEK THREE

Monday

Green coffee bean extract capsules, taken as directed thirty minutes before each meal

Breakfast
Fruit and Nut Granola with low-fat milk (page 76)
Blueberries

Lunch
Large mixed salad (all the veggies you can think of) topped with
   grilled chicken breast, dressed with olive oil and vinegar

Dinner
Scallops baked with lemon and chives
Steamed brown rice
Steamed spinach and baby carrots drizzled with miso dressing

Two snacks (to have between meals if you feel hungry)
Handful of almonds
Low-fat yogurt

Tuesday

Green coffee bean extract capsules, taken as directed thirty
minutes before each meal

Breakfast
Kashi cereal with low-fat milk
Half grapefruit

Lunch
Egg-white omelet with mushrooms, spinach, onions, and tomatoes
Whole-wheat English muffin with slice of low-fat cheddar

Dinner
Braised Chicken with Apricots and Ginger (page 95)
Steamed carrots and broccoli with honey-mustard sauce
Sliced pineapple

Two snacks (to have between meals if you feel hungry)
Guacamole made with ½ mashed avocado and ¼ cup salsa with
   baked tortilla chips
Apple with slice of Swiss cheese

Wednesday

Green coffee bean extract capsules, taken as directed thirty minutes before each meal

Breakfast
Puffed wheat cereal with bananas and milk

Lunch
Vegetarian chili with low-fat cheddar cheese and low-fat sour cream
Green and red peppers

Dinner
Gazpacho soup
Grilled shrimp over your choice of vegetables with lime juice and cilantro

Two snacks (to have between meals if you feel hungry)
Low-fat cottage cheese
Raspberry-Orange Frozen Yogurt (page 74)

Thursday

Green coffee bean extract capsules, taken as directed thirty minutes before each meal

Breakfast
Whole-wheat toast topped with almond butter and banana

Lunch
Veggie burger with slice of cheese and lettuce, tomato, onion, and pickle on a whole-wheat bun
Sliced carrots

Dinner
Miso soup
Salmon-avocado roll
Sashimi

Two snacks (to have between meals if you feel hungry)
Air-popped popcorn
Single-serving container low-fat Greek yogurt

Friday

Green coffee bean extract capsules, taken as directed thirty minutes before each meal

Breakfast
Hard-boiled egg
Fruit salad

Lunch
Big salad with a lot of veggies, grilled salmon, olive oil, vinegar, and oregano
Whole-wheat roll

Dinner
Roasted chicken with fresh garlic and herbs
Asparagus
Cooked quinoa

Two snacks (to have between meals if you feel hungry)
Two squares dark chocolate
Handful of almonds

Saturday

Green coffee bean extract capsules, taken as directed thirty minutes before each meal

Breakfast
Fresh sliced cantaloupe
Pumpkin-Nut Quick Bread (page 78)
Low-fat yogurt
Coffee or tea

Lunch
Carrot-Papaya Coleslaw (page 105)
Lean roast beef sandwich on whole-grain roll with lettuce, spinach, onions, and tomatoes

Dinner
Grilled lean steak with spice rub
Steamed cauliflower
Raspberries

Two snacks (to have between meals if you feel hungry)
Raspberry-Orange frozen yogurt (page 74)
Turnip-Potato Puree (page 101)

Sunday

Green coffee bean extract capsules, taken as directed thirty minutes before each meal

Breakfast
Wheat-bran flakes with blueberries and low-fat milk

Lunch
Small fast-food cheeseburger (ask for extra lettuce, tomato, and onion)
Large garden salad with olive oil and vinegar dressing
Apple

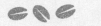 ## DECADENT DESSERTS

Have we convinced you that you'll never feel deprived on this diet? Not yet? Okay, how's this: Here's a list of sweet treats you can enjoy if you are feeling the urge to splurge. Remember: treats, as opposed to snacks, are once-a-day foods, and only if you need them.

- Low-fat hot chocolate
- Gelatin desserts
- Fruit sorbet
- Graham crackers
- Low-fat ice cream
- Fudge pops
- Ice pops
- Low-fat whipped cream
- Pudding (prepared with low-fat milk)

Dinner
Baked pork chop
Wild rice
Steamed broccoli and cauliflower
Watermelon

Two snacks (to have between meals if you feel hungry)
Tropical Fruit Salad (page 79)
Handful almonds

TURN UP THE HEAT ON YOUR MEALS!

In one study, twenty-five participants who spent six weeks sprinkling one half-teaspoon of cayenne pepper on their food raised

GET JIGGY WITH SPICES

Your meals don't have to be monotonous. Experiment with everything on your spice rack to add drama to even the drabbest foods. For example:

- Throw allspice on baked squash.
- Add a kick to any salad with ginger.
- Basil blends well with tomato-sauced dishes.
- Add *oomph* to eggs with chives.
- Introduce a pine-woody flavor to vegetable soup with sage.
- Cinnamon can add a sweetness to any savory dish.
- Add some dill to cottage cheese, or make a dill dip with low-fat sour cream.
- Use rosemary to flavor eggplant, zucchini, stewed tomatoes, or green beans.
- Cardamom adds a unique spicy-sweet taste to lentils.
- Give a punch to vegetable kabobs with mustard seed.
- Add a taste of India to any dish with curry powder or turmeric.

the body's core temperature during digestion, so they burned 10 more calories in the four and a half hours after eating, and ate 70 calories less at their next meal.

Capsaicin, a naturally occurring chemical in peppers that gives them their spicy kick, helps speed up your metabolism and increases calorie burn. Together with your green coffee bean extract, cayenne pepper gives more power to your weight-loss plan. Tabasco and other hot sauces also contain capsaicin.

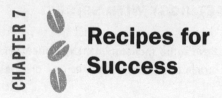

CHAPTER 7

Recipes for Success

BREAKFASTS

Strawberry-Orange Breakfast Smoothie

1 pint fresh strawberries or
   16-ounce package frozen
   strawberries
2 large navel oranges, pared
   and sliced

1 cup nonfat plain yogurt
⅓ cup rice or oat bran
   (available at health-food
   stores)

Place all ingredients in a blender and puree until smooth. Serve over ice.

MAKES: 4 servings

Raspberry-Orange Frozen Yogurt

1 cup orange juice, fresh or from
   concentrate
¼ cup sugar
1 envelope gelatin
One package 12-ounce frozen

raspberries, without syrup,
   thawed
1⅓ cups plain low-fat yogurt
2 teaspoons grated orange zest

1. In a small saucepan, combine the juice, sugar, and gelatin. Heat over very low heat, stirring, until sugar and gelatin have dissolved. Cool to room temperature.

2. Add the raspberries, yogurt, and zest to gelatin mixture. Whisk well to combine.

3. Transfer mixture to a shallow metal baking pan and freeze for 2 hours, then whisk again. Freeze until the mixture is solid, 3 to 4 hours. Before serving, transfer mixture to a food processor. Process until very smooth, about 1 minute.

MAKES: 4 cups

Broiled Grapefruit

1 large grapefruit

Pinch grated nutmeg (optional)

2 teaspoons dark brown sugar

2 teaspoons wheat germ (defatted)

1. Heat broiler. Halve the grapefruit and separate sections with a grapefruit knife. Sprinkle the grapefruit with nutmeg and brown sugar.

2. Broil the grapefruit 2 to 4 inches from heat for 3 to 4 minutes until the edges are browned a bit, the sugar is melted, and the grapefruit is heated through.

3. Sprinkle with the wheat germ and serve immediately.

MAKES: 2 servings

Whole-Grain Buttermilk Pancakes

¼ cup rolled oats (not instant)

½ cup unbleached all-purpose flour

3 tablespoons wheat germ

2 tablespoons sugar

1 tablespoon grated lemon zest

1½ teaspoons baking powder

1 teaspoon baking soda

1 cup buttermilk

1 large egg, separated

1 large egg white

¼ cup pure maple syrup

1. In a food processor, grind the oats to coarse crumbs. Transfer the oats to a medium mixing bowl. Add the flour, wheat germ, sugar, zest, baking powder, and baking soda. Stir well.

2. In a separate bowl, whisk together buttermilk and egg yolk. Pour over the dry ingredients and mix until just combined. In a clean bowl, beat the egg whites until they form soft peaks. Gently fold the egg whites into the batter.

3. Heat griddle or large nonstick skillet over medium heat. Spray with nonstick cooking spray. Drop ¼ cup of the batter onto the hot surface, spreading mixture to 4 to 5 inches. Cook until top is bubbly, about 3 minutes. Flip over and cook until the underside is golden, about 3 more minutes. Continue with the remaining batter, keeping cooked pancakes warm in a low-heated oven.

MAKES: about eight 5-inch pancakes

Fruit and Nut Granola

1 cup old-fashioned rolled oats
½ cup rice bran
½ cup oat bran
½ cup honey
2 tablespoons maple syrup
1 teaspoon vanilla extract
1 cup hazelnuts, coarsely
   chopped

1 cup raw unsalted sunflower
   seeds
½ cup sesame seeds
1 cup wheat germ (defatted)
10 dried apricots, diced
½ cup golden raisins
½ cup pitted dried
   cranberries

1. Preheat oven to 350°F. Toast the rolled oats and brans on a large baking sheet, stirring occasionally, for 10 minutes.

2. Mix the honey, maple syrup, and vanilla in a medium bowl. Add the toasted oat mixture, hazelnuts, sunflower seeds, and sesame seeds. Stir well to coat. Spread the mixture in a thin layer on a baking sheet.

3. Toast the mixture in the oven, stirring every 5 minutes, until well browned, 15 to 20 minutes. Cool completely. Transfer the mixture to a mixing bowl and add the wheat germ and dried fruits. Store in an airtight container. Serve ½ cup servings with ⅓ cup low-fat milk.

MAKES: 16 servings

Oat Bran Bread French Toast with Glazed Apples

Glazed apples (see below for recipe)	¼ teaspoon vanilla extract
1 large egg	Pinch ground allspice
2 large egg whites	1 teaspoon safflower oil
1 tablespoon skim milk	4 slices oat bran bread

1. In a deep plate, beat egg, egg whites, and milk with a fork. Add vanilla and allspice and beat until well blended.

2. Heat oil in a large nonstick skillet over medium heat. Dip bread in the egg mixture and add to skillet. Cook, turning once, until browned on both sides, 3 to 4 minutes each side. Serve hot with glazed apples.

MAKES: 2 servings

Glazed Apples

Pare, core, and thinly slice 2 Granny Smith apples. Heat 1 tablespoon vegetable oil in medium nonstick skillet over medium heat. Add the apples. Stir in ½ cup apple juice, ¼ cup golden raisins, and ⅛ teaspoon pumpkin pie spice.

Cook uncovered, stirring occasionally, until the apples are softened and most of the liquid has evaporated, about 12 minutes.

Potato-Kale Frittata

2 teaspoons olive oil	1 cup grated reduced-fat cheddar cheese
2 cups thinly sliced onion	
3 cups chopped kale	½ cup tomato paste
3 cloves garlic, minced	¼ cup thin strips ham (optional)
1 cup diced, cooked potato	
1 medium tomato, diced	½ teaspoon freshly ground pepper, or to taste
6 eggs or 1½ cups fat-free egg substitute	
	Salt (optional)

1. Preheat broiler.

2. In a 10-inch nonstick ovenproof skillet, heat oil over medium-low heat. Add the onion and cook, stirring, until translucent, 7 to 8 minutes. Add the kale and garlic and cook until the kale is wilted. Tilt the pan so oil covers the sides. Add the potatoes and tomatoes and toss gently.

3. In a small bowl, stir together the egg substitute, cheese, tomato paste, ham, pepper, and salt until well combined. If using whole eggs, beat first, then combine the eggs with the other ingredients.

4. Add egg mixture to the hot skillet and smooth with a spatula. Continue cooking 5 to 6 minutes until the egg is almost set, lifting the sides of the frittata to allow raw egg to run underneath.

5. Place skillet under the broiler to finish cooking, 3 to 4 minutes. Slide frittata onto a plate, cut into wedges, and serve.

MAKES: 4 servings

Pumpkin-Nut Quick Bread

1½ cups unbleached all-purpose flour	½ teaspoon salt
¼ cup whole-wheat flour	½ teaspoon ground allspice
½ cup chopped walnuts	½ teaspoon ground cinnamon
½ cup raisins	¼ teaspoon ground cloves
⅓ cup sugar	¼ teaspoon grated nutmeg
⅓ cup wheat germ	1 cup pumpkin puree, canned or homemade
2½ teaspoons baking powder	1 large egg
1 teaspoon baking soda	1 large egg white
2 teaspoons grated orange zest	1 teaspoon pure vanilla extract

1. Preheat oven to 350°F. Spray a 9 × 5-inch loaf pan with nonstick cooking spray. Sprinkle the pan with flour. Shake off the excess.

2. In a large bowl, combine flours, walnuts, raisins, sugar, wheat germ, baking powder, baking soda, zest, salt, and spices. Stir well. In a separate bowl, whisk together the pumpkin puree, egg, egg white, and vanilla.

3. Pour the liquid ingredients over the dry ingredients. Stir just until blended. Pour the mixture into the prepared pan.

4. Bake 1 hour 25 minutes, until a toothpick inserted in the center comes out clean. Cool in the pan on a wire rack.

MAKES: 10 servings

SALADS AND SOUPS

White Bean and Broccoli Salad

2 cups broccoli florets steamed crisp-tender

2 cups cooked small white beans, or one 16-ounce can, rinsed and drained

⅓ cup diced roasted red pepper

2 tablespoons olive oil

1 tablespoon fresh lemon juice

1 clove garlic, minced

Pinch each salt and red pepper flakes

Stir together all the ingredients in a medium bowl. Serve at room temperature.

MAKES: 2 servings

Tropical Fruit Salad

1 mango, peeled and cubed

1 cup cubed cantaloupe

1 papaya, peeled, seeded, and cubed

2 kiwis, peeled, halved, and sliced ½ inch thick

1 lime, sectioned

½ teaspoon grated fresh ginger

1 tablespoon chopped fresh mint leaves

In large bowl, combine all fruits and mint. Toss gently.

MAKES: 4 servings

Pasta, Broccoli, and Basil Salad

12 ounces spiral pasta
4 cups broccoli florets
2 red bell peppers, seeded and thinly slivered
¼ cup red wine vinegar
½ cup crumbled feta cheese

1 tablespoon extra-virgin olive oil
¼ teaspoon freshly ground black pepper
1 cup (packed) fresh basil leaves, chopped

1. Cook the pasta according to the package directions. Add the broccoli to the pasta in boiling water for the last 3 minutes of cooking. Drain the pasta and broccoli, reserving ¼ cup of the cooking liquid.

2. In a large bowl, combine the red peppers, vinegar, feta, oil, and black pepper.

3. Toss the warm pasta, broccoli, and reserved cooking liquid with the red pepper mixture. Toss with the basil and let stand for 30 minutes before serving.

MAKES: 4 servings

Sweet Potato–Orange Soup

¼ cup safflower oil
3 onions, chopped
2 medium sweet potatoes, peeled and grated
3 carrots, peeled and grated
2 stalks celery, chopped
6 cups chicken broth (no salt added)
1 cup water
One 16-ounce can white beans,

rinsed and drained, or 2 cups cooked beans
3 large navel oranges, pared and sectioned
½ teaspoon salt or to taste
¼ teaspoon freshly ground pepper or to taste
Pinch grated orange peel
One 12-ounce can evaporated low-fat milk
Chopped fresh parsley for garnish

1. Heat the oil in a large Dutch oven over medium heat. Add the onions and cook for 5 minutes, stirring often. Add the remaining vegetables, chicken broth, and water. Raise the heat and bring to a boil. Lower heat to medium and simmer the soup for 15 minutes.

2. Remove the pot from the heat and add the beans, oranges, salt, pepper, and orange peel. Working in batches, puree in a food processor until smooth.

3. Put the soup back in the pot and put the pot back on the heat. Add milk and cook over medium heat until the soup is just heated through. Taste the soup and adjust the seasonings. Garnish with parsley and serve hot.

MAKES: 8 servings

Oriental Chicken and Bean Salad

1 chicken breast, skinned, boned, and split	3 tablespoons safflower oil
2 cups cooked garbanzo beans or one 16-ounce can, rinsed and drained	2 tablespoons balsamic vinegar
2 cups cooked black-eyed peas, or one 16-ounce can, rinsed and drained	2 tablespoons minced coriander leaves
2 carrots, peeled, halved lengthwise, and sliced	1 teaspoon sesame oil
2 scallions, minced	1 teaspoon soy sauce (low-sodium)
	2 teaspoons minced fresh ginger
	Dash hot red pepper sauce

1. Poach the chicken breast, beginning in cold water, over medium heat in a medium saucepan, for 5 to 7 minutes after water comes to a simmer, until cooked through. Remove the chicken from the pan and cool. When cool enough to handle, cut the chicken into thin strips.

2. Stir the chicken together with the remaining ingredients in a medium bowl. Serve at room temperature.

MAKES: 6 servings

Split Pea Soup

3 tablespoons safflower oil	1 pound green split
3 medium onions, chopped	peas
3 carrots, chopped	1 small bunch parsley
3 celery stalks, trimmed and	1 teaspoon salt
chopped	½ teaspoon freshly ground
8 cups water or as needed	pepper

1. Heat the oil in a large Dutch oven over medium heat. Add the onions, carrots, and celery. Cook, stirring occasionally, for 10 minutes.

2. Add the remaining ingredients. Bring the soup to a boil over medium-high heat. Reduce heat, stirring occasionally, and simmer partially covered over medium heat for 40 to 45 minutes. Thin the soup with more water if necessary.

3. Working in batches, carefully pass the soup through a food mill or puree in a food processor. Taste the soup and adjust the seasonings. Serve hot.

MAKES: 6 servings

Shrimp and Black Bean Salad

Lime-Ginger vinaigrette (page 83)	10 scallions, minced
	½ cup minced fresh coriander
3 cups cooked or canned black beans, drained and rinsed	1 bunch radishes, trimmed and sliced thin
2 small heads romaine, shredded	2 carrots, peeled and sliced thin
1 small bunch arugula, large stems removed	Juice of 2 limes
1 yellow bell pepper, seeded and diced	1 pound cooked medium shrimp, shelled and deveined
1 red bell pepper, seeded and diced	¼ cup toasted pine nuts

1. Place the beans in a medium bowl and toss with vinaigrette.

2. Toss together all the remaining ingredients except the shrimp and pine nuts.

3. Place the greens and vegetables on 6 dinner plates. Top with the bean mixture. Top each plate with shrimp and pine nuts. Serve immediately.

MAKES: 6 servings

Lime-Ginger Vinaigrette

Whisk together ½ cup chicken broth, ¼ cup lime juice, 3 tablespoons extra-virgin olive oil, 1 tablespoon minced fresh ginger, ½ teaspoon each ground coriander, salt, and hot red pepper sauce to taste.

Tuna and Black-Eyed Pea Salad

2 cups cooked black-eyed peas or one 16-ounce can, rinsed and drained	3 tablespoons fresh lime juice
	2 tablespoons safflower oil
6½-ounce can tuna, packed in water	1 tablespoon minced fresh basil
3 scallions, minced	¼ teaspoon grated lime peel
	⅛ teaspoon cayenne pepper

Stir together all the ingredients in a medium bowl. Serve at room temperature or chilled.

MAKES: 2 servings

Vegetable Lentil Soup

¼ cup extra-virgin olive oil
2 onions, diced
1 red bell pepper, seeded and
    diced
1 carrot, peeled and sliced
1 clove garlic, peeled and
    minced
2 small zucchini, trimmed and
    grated
3 cups chicken broth
2 cups water or as needed
½ pound lentils

1 cup canned crushed
    tomatoes
1 bay leaf
½ teaspoon thyme, dried
½ teaspoon oregano, dried
½ teaspoon salt
½ teaspoon cayenne pepper
1 cup cooked brown rice
1 tablespoon balsamic vinegar
    or to taste
Shredded fresh basil for
    garnish

1. Heat the oil over medium heat in a Dutch oven. Add the onion, pepper, carrot, and garlic. Cook, stirring occasionally, for 10 minutes. Add the zucchini and cook for 5 minutes longer.

2. Add the broth, water, lentils, tomatoes, and bay leaf. Bring to a boil over medium-high heat. Reduce the heat to medium and simmer partially covered for 15 minutes.

3. Add the herbs, salt, and pepper and simmer for 15 minutes longer. Add the rice. Taste and adjust seasonings. Remove from heat and add vinegar. Serve hot, garnished with shredded basil.

MAKES: 6 servings

Sliced Steak and Roasted Tomato Salad

12 ounces flank steak, trimmed

Salt, to taste

Freshly ground pepper, to taste

12 plum tomatoes, roasted

1 cup sliced red onion

1 red bell pepper, seeded and slivered

1 orange, sectioned

2 tablespoons chopped fresh rosemary leaves

1 tablespoon orange juice, fresh or from concentrate

2 teaspoons extra-virgin olive oil

1 clove garlic, peeled and minced

3 cups arugula leaves

1. Preheat broiler.

2. Season steak with salt and black pepper. Broil the steak, 4 to 6 inches from the heat, to desired doneness. Allow the meat to rest for 5 minutes. Slice thinly against the grain.

3. In a large bowl, combine tomatoes, onion, red pepper, orange, rosemary, orange juice, olive oil, garlic, black pepper, and salt. Toss gently until combined.

4. Add the arugula to the mixture. Toss gently. Arrange on plates along with the steak. Serve promptly.

MAKES: 4 servings

Summer Tomato Salad

1½ pounds ripe tomatoes, cut in wedges

¼ cup thinly sliced red onion

½ cup packed fresh basil leaves, shredded

3 tablespoons red wine vinegar

1 tablespoon extra-virgin olive oil

¼ teaspoon freshly ground black pepper

Salt to taste

1 teaspoon chopped garlic (optional)

1. In a large bowl, combine tomatoes, onion, and basil. Set aside.

2. In a small bowl, whisk together vinegar, oil, pepper, salt, and garlic (if using). Gently toss the dressing with the tomato

mixture. Cover with plastic wrap and set aside for 1 hour, stirring once. Do not refrigerate. Serve at room temperature.

MAKES: 4 servings

Chicken–Wild Rice Salad with Mango and Ginger

5 cups low-sodium chicken broth, or water

1 cup wild rice, rinsed and drained

2 cups shredded, cooked chicken breast

2 large ripe mangoes, peeled and diced

1 medium tomato, diced

1 red bell pepper, seeded and diced

1 cup diced cucumber

½ cup thinly sliced scallions

2 tablespoons chopped walnuts

⅓ cup orange juice, fresh or from concentrate

2 tablespoons extra-virgin olive oil

1 teaspoon distilled white vinegar

1½ teaspoons grated fresh ginger

½ teaspoon freshly ground black pepper

Salt to taste (optional)

1. In a medium saucepan, bring the broth or water to a boil. Stir in the wild rice, reduce heat to low, and simmer, uncovered, until tender, about 45 minutes. Drain well and cool the rice to room temperature.

2. In a large bowl, combine the rice, chicken, mango, tomato, red pepper, cucumber, scallions, and walnuts.

3. In a separate bowl, combine the orange juice, oil, vinegar, ginger, pepper, and salt. Toss with the mango mixture.

MAKES: 4 servings

Fennel and Orange Salad with Parsley and Olives

1 fennel bulb, halved and thinly
  sliced
4 navel oranges, sectioned
½ cup packed Italian flat-leaf
  parsley leaves, chopped
2 tablespoons orange juice,
  fresh or from concentrate

4 teaspoons extra-virgin olive oil
8 cured green olives, pitted and
  slivered
1 teaspoon grated orange zest
¼ teaspoon freshly ground
  black pepper
Salt to taste (optional)

In a medium bowl, combine all of the ingredients. Toss well.

MAKES: 4 servings

MAIN COURSES

Linguine with Shrimp

6 tablespoons extra-virgin olive oil
2 small onions, sliced in thin rings
1 small red bell pepper,
  seeded and diced
1 small yellow bell pepper,
  seeded and diced
2 cloves garlic, peeled and
  minced
1 pound linguine, preferably
  whole wheat or oat bran
1½ cups broccoli florets

One 16-ounce can garbanzo
  beans, drained and rinsed
  or 2 cups cooked beans
1 pound cooked medium shrimp,
  shelled and deveined
¼ cup minced fresh parsley
2 tablespoons toasted pine nuts
1 tablespoon drained capers
¼ teaspoon salt
¼ teaspoon crushed red pepper
  flakes

1. Heat oil in a large skillet over medium heat. Add the onions and cook, stirring occasionally, for 5 minutes until lightly browned. Add the red and yellow peppers and garlic and cook for 2 minutes longer, stirring frequently.

2. Meanwhile, cook the linguine according to the package directions, adding the broccoli to the boiling water for the last 3 minutes of cooking. Drain and keep warm

3. Add the garbanzo beans to the skillet and cook 3 minutes longer, stirring frequently. Add the cooked pasta, shrimp, parsley, pine nuts, and capers. Season to taste with salt and crushed red pepper flakes. Toss to mix and serve hot.

MAKES: 6 servings

Tilapia in Spicy Tomato Sauce

2 teaspoons extra-virgin olive oil
1 cup chopped onion
2 cloves garlic, peeled and minced
¼ cup dry white wine
One 28-ounce can whole plum tomatoes in juice, coarsely chopped, juice reserved

1 cup water
1 teaspoon grated orange zest
¼ to ½ teaspoon hot pepper flakes
1 sprig fresh rosemary
Four 6-ounce tilapia fillets

1. In a large nonstick skillet, heat oil over medium-high heat. Add the onion and cook, stirring until tender, 4 to 5 minutes. Add the garlic and cook 1 minute. Add the wine and continue cooking, stirring until the wine evaporates.

2. Add tomatoes and juice, water, zest, pepper flakes, and whole rosemary sprig. Simmer until sauce has thickened, 15 minutes.

3. Nestle the fish fillets in the tomato sauce. Partially cover and cook until fish is just cooked through, 4 to 8 minutes, depending on thickness. Serve fillets topped with sauce, first removing rosemary sprig.

MAKES: 4 servings

Falafel

One 20-ounce can white fava
   beans or garbanzo beans,
   rinsed and drained, or 2 cups
   cooked beans
4 scallions, thinly sliced
¼ cup minced fresh parsley
4 cloves garlic, peeled and
   minced
1 tablespoon ground cumin

1 tablespoon ground coriander
1½ teaspoons baking powder
¼ teaspoon salt
¼ teaspoon cayenne pepper
¼ teaspoon grated lemon
   peel
2 to 3 tablespoons toasted
   wheat germ (defatted)
1 tablespoon safflower oil

1. Puree the beans in a food processor. Add the scallions, parsley, garlic, cumin, coriander, baking powder, salt, cayenne pepper, and lemon peel. Pulse until well blended. Place the mixture in a small bowl and stir in the wheat germ until the mixture is slightly stiff. Let sit covered in a refrigerator for at least 30 minutes.

2. Heat oil in a large nonstick skillet. Shape the falafel mixture into 8 patties, about 2½ × ½ inch. Cook the patties until browned on both sides, turning once, about 4 minutes each side.

MAKES: 4 servings

Chicken Chili

1 tablespoon safflower oil

2 small onions, diced

2 small carrots, peeled, halved lengthwise, and sliced thin

1 clove garlic, peeled and minced

1½ teaspoons ground cumin seed

½ teaspoon ground coriander seed

½ teaspoon marjoram

¼ teaspoon grated lime peel

1 whole chicken breast, skinned, boned, split, and cut into thin strips

2 cups cooked small white beans or one 16-ounce can, drained and rinsed

½ cup chicken broth, or as needed

One 4-ounce can chopped roasted green chilis, drained

3 scallions, minced

¼ cup diced roasted red peppers (fresh or jarred)

Salt and cayenne pepper to taste

Lime wedges for garnish

1. Heat oil in a large skillet over medium heat. Add the onions, carrots, and garlic. Cook for 5 minutes, stirring occasionally. Add the cumin, ground coriander, marjoram, and lime peel. Cook, stirring constantly, until very fragrant, about 1 to 2 minutes.

2. Add the chicken and cook, stirring frequently, for about 4 minutes, until chicken is cooked through. Add the beans, chicken broth, and roasted green chilis. Cook, stirring occasionally, until slightly thickened, about 10 minutes. Add the salt and cayenne pepper to taste, serve with lime wedges as a garnish.

MAKES: 4 servings

Chicken Burgers

2 whole chicken breasts, skinned, boned, and cut into large chunks
2 ounces Canadian bacon, diced
8 dried apricots, diced
5 tablespoons oat bran, divided
2 tablespoons old-fashioned oatmeal

1 large egg or equivalent egg substitute
4 scallions, minced
¼ cup parsley, minced
Pinch each salt and freshly ground pepper
Pinch grated lemon peel
1 tablespoon safflower oil

1. Trim the fat from the chicken. Place the chicken in the bowl of a food processor and add the Canadian bacon, apricots, 3 tablespoons oat bran, oatmeal, and egg. Process until ground and well blended.

2. Remove the chicken mixture from the processor and place in a medium bowl. Stir in scallions, parsley, salt, pepper, and lemon peel; mix completely.

3. Shape the mixture into 4 oval patties, about ¾ inch thick. Coat with the remaining 2 tablespoons oat bran.

4. Heat oil in a large nonstick skillet over medium heat. Add the patties and cook until browned, about 5 minutes each side. Serve hot.

MAKES: 4 servings

Grilled Salmon with Spinach and White Beans

⅓ cup mango chutney
¼ cup plain nonfat yogurt
One 16-ounce can small white beans, rinsed and drained, or 2 cups cooked white beans
Two 4-ounce salmon steaks
1 tablespoon safflower oil, divided

3 cups shredded, well-cleaned spinach
Pinch each salt and freshly ground pepper
1 tablespoon minced fresh parsley or coriander leaves

1. Puree the chutney and yogurt in a food processor. Place the puree in a small bowl and stir in beans. Set aside at room temperature.

2. Brush the salmon steaks with 1 teaspoon oil and grill over charcoal, or in a grill pan for 4 minutes or more on each side, depending on the thickness, until cooked as desired.

3. Toss the spinach with the remaining oil, salt, and pepper. Place the spinach on dinner plates and top with the salmon and then the bean mixture. Sprinkle with parsley or coriander. Serve immediately.

MAKES: 2 servings

Pork Medallions with Black Beans

2 tablespoons plus 1 teaspoon safflower oil

6 scallions, minced

2 teaspoons minced fresh ginger

Two 16-ounce cans black beans, rinsed and drained, or 4 cups cooked black beans

One 16-ounce can crushed tomatoes

One 4-ounce can chopped roasted green chilis

Four 3-ounce pork medallions, slightly pounded and trimmed of all fat

Pinch each salt and fresh ground pepper

2 tablespoons minced fresh coriander leaves

Plain nonfat yogurt for garnish

1. Heat 2 tablespoons oil in a medium skillet over medium heat. Add the scallions and ginger and cook, stirring frequently, for about 2 minutes, until very fragrant.

2. Add the beans, tomatoes, and chilis. Cook, stirring occasionally, for 10 minutes, until thickened.

3. Meanwhile, heat the remaining oil in a large nonstick skillet over medium heat. Add the pork and sauté until cooked through, about 3 minutes each side. Season with salt and pepper.

4. Place the pork medallions on dinner plates and top with the black bean mixture. Garnish with coriander and yogurt and serve immediately.

MAKES: 4 servings

Shepherd's Pie with Sweet Potato Topping

1 pound Idaho potatoes, scrubbed	8 canned tomatoes, roasted, or ½ cup soaked sun-dried
1 pound sweet potatoes, scrubbed	tomatoes, chopped
2 teaspoons safflower oil	1 tablespoon chopped fresh rosemary leaves
1 cup chopped onion	1 teaspoon chopped fresh
1 pound lean ground beef	thyme leaves
1½ cups reduced-sodium beef broth, canned or homemade	2 cups packed chopped fresh spinach (6 ounces)

1. Preheat oven to 400°F.

2. Bake Idaho and sweet potatoes until soft, 45 to 60 minutes. Remove the potatoes from the oven, reducing the oven temperature to 375°F. When potatoes are cool enough to handle, peel. In a large bowl, combine the potatoes and mash with a potato masher. Set aside.

3. In a large nonstick skillet, heat oil over medium high heat. Add the onion and cook, stirring until it begins to brown, 5 to 6 minutes. Reduce the heat to medium. Add the beef and continue cooking, stirring, until beef is no longer pink. Add broth, tomatoes, rosemary, and thyme. Simmer for 10 minutes.

4. Add the spinach and cook, stirring until spinach is just wilted. Remove the skillet from the heat.

5. Transfer the mixture to a 6-cup baking dish and spoon mashed potatoes over the top of the mixture, covering it completely. Bake until top is golden, about 45 minutes.

MAKES: 4 servings

Tomato-Stuffed Pork Tenderloin with Roasted Poblano Sauce

4 poblano peppers, roasted

¼ cup water

1 tablespoon fresh lemon juice

3 teaspoons extra-virgin olive oil, divided

Salt to taste

Two 8-ounce pork tenderloins

2 cloves garlic, peeled and minced

¼ teaspoon salt

1 tablespoon chopped fresh thyme leaves

14 tomatoes, canned or fresh, roasted

1. Preheat grill or broiler.

2. In a food processor, combine peppers, water, lemon juice, 2 teaspoons of the oil, and salt to taste. Puree until smooth. Set aside.

3. Slice tenderloins lengthwise almost all the way through, open on a work surface. Pound tenderloins gently, without breaking through the meat, until ⅛ to ¼ inch thick. Rub each tenderloin with the remaining ½ teaspoon olive oil.

4. Chop garlic with ¼ teaspoon salt, pressing it into a smooth paste with the side of knife. Spread the garlic on the tenderloins and sprinkle with thyme. Line 7 tomatoes along the long edge of each tenderloin. Roll up the tenderloin tightly, securing ends and middle with toothpicks.

5. Grill or broil the pork, turning gradually, until browned on all sides and cooked through, 18 to 20 minutes. Remove from the heat, remove the toothpicks, and let rest for 5 minutes. Cut, against the grain, into ¼-inch slices and serve with poblano sauce.

MAKES: 4 servings

Braised Chicken with Apricots and Ginger

8 small chicken thighs, skin and excess fat removed

1 teaspoon freshly ground black pepper

½ teaspoon salt

2 teaspoons safflower oil

1½ cups chopped onion

1 tablespoon grated fresh ginger

2 cloves garlic, peeled and minced

Zest of one 2×1-inch orange peel

2 teaspoons ground cardamom

1 teaspoon ground turmeric

¾ teaspoon ground cloves

1 cup low-sodium chicken broth, canned or homemade, or water

1 cup dried apricots (6 ounces), sliced in ⅛- to ¼-inch strips

1. Preheat oven to 350°F. Sprinkle chicken thighs with pepper and salt.

2. In a Dutch oven, heat oil over medium heat. Add the onion and cook until translucent. Add the ginger, garlic, orange zest, cardamom, turmeric, and cloves and continue cooking 1 more minute. Add the broth or water and apricots. Remove from heat.

3. Nestle chicken thighs in the apricot mixture. Cover the pot with foil, then with the lid to create an air-tight seal. Place the pot in the oven and cook until the chicken is tender, about 90 minutes.

MAKES: 4 servings

DESSERTS

Oranges with Strawberry Sauce

3 navel oranges

½ cup hulled and sliced strawberries (or unsweetened frozen strawberries)

1 tablespoon superfine sugar or to taste

1 teaspoon orange-flavored liqueur

1. Cut peel and white pith from all oranges, then cut orange sections away from membranes with a small sharp knife over a small bowl to catch juices; reserve 2 tablespoons juice. Grate and set aside large pinch of orange peel.

2. Place strawberries in the bowl of a food processor with the orange peel and juice, sugar, and orange liqueur. Process until smooth.

3. Transfer the orange sections with a slotted spoon to 2 chilled dessert bowls. Spoon the strawberry sauce over the oranges and garnish with strawberries, candied violets, and mint sprigs, if desired.

Almond Angel Food Cake with Mango Puree

6 large egg whites	½ cup finely ground almonds
½ teaspoon cream of tartar	1 teaspoon pure vanilla extract
¼ teaspoon salt	½ teaspoon almond extract
½ cup plus 1 tablespoon super- fine sugar	⅓ cup water
	2 tablespoons granulated sugar
½ cup sifted cake flour	3 ripe mangoes

1. Preheat oven to 325°F.

2. In a large bowl, beat egg whites until frothy. Add the cream of tartar and salt, and continue beating until soft peaks form. Continue beating while gradually adding the superfine sugar. Beat until stiff.

3. Sift 2 tablespoons of the flour over egg whites. Gently fold into the mixture. Repeat with the remaining flour, 2 tablespoons at a time. Fold in the nuts, then the vanilla and almond extracts.

4. Transfer mixture to a 9-inch tube pan. Bake until the cake pulls away from the sides of the pan, about 45 minutes. Invert pan onto a rack and cool thoroughly before removing the cake.

5. In a small saucepan, combine water and granulated sugar. Heat until the sugar is dissolved. Increase the heat and boil until just beginning to color, about 6 minutes. Do not stir the syrup.

6. Remove the mango pulp from the skin and discard the pit. Transfer the pulp to a food processor. Process the pulp until smooth. Add the sugar syrup and process to mix. Serve with the cake.

MAKES: 6 servings

Strawberries in Balsamic Vinegar

2 pints strawberries

¼ cup honey

2 tablespoons balsamic vinegar

Hull the strawberries and cut them in half. Combine the berries and honey in a medium bowl and let stand for 30 minutes before serving. Sprinkle with vinegar and gently toss to blend. Serve immediately.

MAKES: 6 servings

Oatmeal Cookies

1¼ cup old-fashioned oatmeal

½ cup all-purpose flour

½ cup wheat germ

½ cup sesame seeds

¼ cup oat bran

¼ cup golden raisins

¼ cup minced dried peaches

¼ cup finely chopped pitted prunes

1 teaspoon baking powder

½ teaspoon salt

½ cup margarine

½ cup dark brown sugar

¼ cup sugar

1 large egg or equivalent egg substitute

1 teaspoon vanilla extract

1 teaspoon grated lemon peel

1. Heat oven to 375°F. In a medium bowl combine the oatmeal, flour, wheat germ, sesame seeds, oat bran, golden raisins, peaches, prunes, baking powder, and salt. Stir until well mixed.

2. Cream the margarine and sugars in a large mixing bowl. Add the egg and blend. Add the vanilla and lemon peel and mix well. Add the dry ingredients and mix well. If the dough is dry, add 1 to 2 tablespoons of water.

3. Drop the dough by tablespoonfuls onto nonstick baking sheets and flatten slightly. Bake 10 to 12 minutes, until the cookies are golden and edges are browning. Cool for 3 minutes on the baking sheets, then remove the cookies with a spatula, and continue to cool the cookies on a rack.

MAKES: 2 dozen cookies

Papaya Sorbet

2 large ripe papayas   2 tablespoons honey
Juice of 2 limes

1. Pare and seed the papaya, and coarsely chop. Put the papaya and remaining ingredients in the bowl of a food processor and puree until smooth.

2. Freeze in an ice-cream maker according to the manufacturer's directions, about 30 minutes. Remove from the canister and store in the freezer until ready to serve. This is best served the same day it's prepared.

3. If you don't have an ice-cream maker, pour the papaya mixture into ice cube trays or a freezer container. Cover and freeze until mixture forms a 2-inch frame of ice around perimeter of the pan, about 1½ to 2 hours. Remove from the freezer. Scrape ice from the sides of the container and stir with a whisk, or pour into a bowl and use an electric mixer to break up the ice crystals and incorporate air into the mixture. Return to the freezer for 30 to 50 minutes and repeat the above. If you want a very smooth sorbet, you may have to repeat the process again, but it will require less freezing time.

MAKES: 4 servings

Frozen Banana Dessert

2 bananas

1 cup hulled and sliced
   strawberries, chilled

½ chilled papaya,
   pared, seeded, and diced

2 teaspoons toasted defatted
   wheat germ (optional)

2 whole strawberries and mint
   sprigs for garnish

1. Peel and quarter bananas. Place them in a sealed plastic bag in the freezer overnight.

2. Just before serving, place bananas and strawberries in the bowl of a food processor. Process until creamy. spoon the fruit mixture into serving bowls. Top with diced papaya and wheat germ. Garnish with strawberries and mint. Serve immediately.

MAKES: 2 servings

Cantaloupe Granita

1 cup water

¼ cup sugar

4 cups cantaloupe chunks

1 tablespoon fresh lime juice

1. In a 1-quart saucepan, heat water and sugar over medium heat until the sugar is dissolved. Transfer to a food processor. Add the cantaloupe and lime juice. Process the mixture until smooth.

2. Transfer the mixture to a shallow metal baking pan and freeze for 2 hours, stirring the mixture every 30 minutes. Return to a food processor and process until smooth. Transfer to a covered plastic container and keep frozen until ready to serve.

MAKES: 4 servings

Ginger Baked Apples

2 Golden Delicious apples,
cored from stem end, bottom
intact
2 teaspoons minced crystallized
ginger

2 cinnamon sticks
¼ cup unsweetened apple
juice
Pinch ground allspice

1. Heat oven to 350°F.
2. Place the apples stem up in a 9-inch glass pie dish. Place 1 teaspoon ginger and 1 cinnamon stick in each apple. Mix apple juice and allspice, then pour into center of each apple.
3. Bake until tender when pierced with a fork, 35 to 40 minutes. Serve warm.

MAKES: 2 servings

SIDE DISHES AND SNACKS

Baked Sweet Potato Fries

Four 8-ounce sweet potatoes,
scrubbed
1 teaspoon extra-virgin olive oil

⅛ teaspoon cayenne
pepper
Salt to taste (optional)

1. Preheat the oven to 450°F.
2. Cut the unpeeled potatoes lengthwise into ⅓ inch thick slices, then cut into sticks. In a large bowl, combine oil and cayenne pepper. Add the potatoes and toss until well coated.
3. Transfer the potatoes to a baking sheet coated with nonstick cooking spray. Bake 15 minutes, turn and continue cooking until golden, 15 to 20 minutes. Sprinkle with salt if using.

MAKES: 4 servings

Whole-Wheat Garlic Chips

½ cup whole-wheat flour
½ cup all-purpose flour
¼ cup wheat germ
3 cloves garlic, peeled and
   minced
2 teaspoons sugar
1 teaspoon baking powder

½ teaspoon freshly ground
   pepper
½ teaspoon salt
¼ cup plain low-fat yogurt
1 tablespoon safflower oil
⅓ cup very cold water, or as
   needed

1. Preheat the oven to 350°F. Spray a baking sheet with non-stick cooking spray.

2. In a large bowl, combine flours, wheat germ, garlic, sugar, baking powder, pepper, and salt.

3. In a small bowl, combine yogurt and oil. Add the yogurt mixture to the flour mixture, stirring. Gradually add the water until mixture forms a dough. Knead slightly until the dough forms a mass.

4. Roll out the dough until ¹⁄₁₆ inch thick. Cut the dough with a knife or pastry cutter into 2-inch squares. Halve squares into triangles.

5. Place triangles on the prepared baking sheet. Bake until golden brown, about 10 minutes. Cool on rack.

MAKES: about 50 chips

Turnip-Potato Puree

3 purple-top turnips
   (1½ pounds), peeled and cut
   into 1-inch pieces
2 large all-purpose potatoes
   (1¼ pounds), peeled
   and cut into 1-inch
   pieces
¾ cup packed fresh Italian

flat-leaf parsley leaves,
   chopped
2 tablespoons sour cream
   or greek yogurt
½ teaspoon freshly ground
   black pepper
⅛ teaspoon grated nutmeg
Salt to taste

1. In a steamer basket, steam the turnips over 1 inch of gently boiling water until tender, 10 to 15 minutes. Meanwhile, in a separate saucepan of boiling water, boil potatoes until tender, 10 to 15 minutes. Drain both well.

2. Transfer the turnips and potatoes to a food processor. Add the parsley, sour cream, pepper, nutmeg, and salt. Puree until smooth.

MAKES: 4 servings

Oat Groats with Carrots and Parsley

2 cups water or chicken stock

1 cup whole oat groats

½ teaspoon salt

1 tablespoon safflower oil

1 medium onion, diced

1 carrot, peeled and grated

1 clove garlic, peeled and minced

2 tablespoons minced fresh parsley

Salt and freshly ground pepper to taste

1. Combine water, oat groats, and salt in a heavy medium-size saucepan. Bring to a boil over high heat. Reduce heat, and simmer slowly, stirring occasionally, for 45 minutes or until done. Rinse if desired and drain. Set aside in a bowl.

2. Meanwhile, heat oil in a medium skillet. Add the onion and cook, stirring frequently, until the onion is soft, about 4 to 5 minutes. Add the carrot and garlic and cook, stirring constantly, for 2 minutes. Add the carrot mixture to the cooked oat groats with parsley, salt, and pepper and serve hot.

MAKES: 4 servings

Brown Rice

1 cup brown rice
2 cups water

Pinch salt

Bring all the ingredients to a boil. Boil, covered, for 10 minutes. Turn off the heat and let sit at least 3 hours or all day. Before serving just gently reheat the rice.

MAKES: 4 servings

Carrots with Cumin

8 medium carrots, peeled, cut
  into triangle shapes (1 inch
  thick at widest parts)
¼ cup chicken broth

¼ teaspoon ground cumin
  seeds
Pinch each salt and freshly
  ground pepper

1. Cook the carrots in a medium saucepan, covered, in a lot of boiling water until crisp-tender, 3 to 4 minutes. Drain well.

2. Just before serving, put carrots in a medium nonstick skillet with the remaining ingredients. Cook, stirring frequently over medium heat until heated through, about 2 minutes. Serve immediately.

MAKES: 4 servings

Braised Red Cabbage

2 tablespoons safflower
  oil
1 medium onion, minced
½ small head red cabbage,
  shredded
1 Golden Delicious apple,
  pared, cored, and finely
  diced
½ cup chicken broth

¼ cup plus 5 tablespoons dry
  white wine
2 teaspoons fresh lime juice
1 teaspoon Dijon mustard
½ teaspoon sugar
¼ teaspoon grated lime peel
¼ teaspoon freshly ground
  pepper
¼ teaspoon salt

1. Heat oil in medium nonstick skillet over medium heat. Add the onion and sauté, stirring occasionally, until softened, about 4 minutes.

2. Add remaining ingredients and cook, stirring occasionally, until cabbage is softened and most of the cooking liquid is absorbed, about 15 minutes. Serve hot.

MAKES: 2 servings

Brussels Sprouts with Shallots

1 tablespoon safflower
  oil
3 shallots, minced

1 pound Brussels sprouts,
  trimmed and shredded
Salt and freshly ground pepper

Heat oil in large nonstick skillet over medium heat. Add shallots; cook until softened, about 3 minutes. Add sprouts and cook, stirring often, over medium-high heat for 5 to 7 minutes, until crisp-tender. Season to taste with salt and pepper and serve hot.

MAKES: 6 servings

Parsley–White Bean Dip

3 cups cooked cannellini or
  other white beans, or
  canned, drained and rinsed
1 cup packed Italian fresh flat-
  leaf parsley leaves, blanched
  quickly in boiling water
1 tablespoon extra-virgin

  olive oil
1 clove garlic, peeled and minced
½ teaspoon grated lemon zest
½ teaspoon freshly ground
  black pepper
Salt to taste
Water as needed

In the bowl of a food processor, combine beans, parsley, lemon juice, rosemary, olive oil, garlic, zest, pepper, and salt. Process the mixture until smooth, adding water 1 tablespoon at a time if necessary.

MAKES: 6 servings

Carrot-Papaya Coleslaw

2 cups shredded green cabbage

2 medium carrots, grated

1 red bell pepper, seeded and thinly slivered

1 papaya, peeled, seeded, and slivered

¼ cup reduced-fat mayonnaise

⅓ cup packed fresh cilantro leaves, chopped

2 tablespoons fresh lemon juice

½ to 1 roasted jalapeño pepper, finely minced

1 clove garlic, peeled and minced

¼ teaspoon freshly ground black pepper

1. In a large bowl, combine cabbage, carrots, red pepper, and papaya. Set aside.

2. In a small bowl, combine mayonnaise, cilantro, lemon juice, jalapeño, garlic, and black pepper. Add to the cabbage mixture. Toss well.

MAKES: 4 servings

Strawberry Yogurt and Fruit

One 10-ounce package thawed frozen strawberries

1 cup plain nonfat yogurt

3 navel oranges, pared, and

white pith removed, sectioned

1 papaya, pared, seeded, and cut into ½-inch dice

2 bananas, sliced

1. Puree the strawberries with their syrup in a food processor or blender. Place in a small bowl and stir in the yogurt.

2. Gently combine the oranges, papaya, and bananas. Evenly divide half of the strawberry yogurt in the bottoms of 4 goblets. Top with fruit and add the remaining yogurt. Serve immediately.

MAKES: 4 servings

Tropical Citrus Shake

1 papaya peeled, seeded, and cut into chunks
1 persimmon, peeled and cored
¼ cup orange juice, fresh or from concentrate
¼ cup fresh lime juice
1½ teaspoons grated fresh ginger
6 ice cubes

Combine papaya, persimmon, juices, ginger, and ice in a blender or food processor. Pulse until well combined and the ice is crushed. Serve in tall glasses.

MAKES: 2 servings

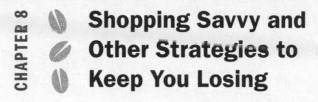

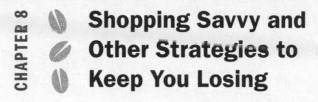 **CHAPTER 8** **Shopping Savvy and Other Strategies to Keep You Losing**

I n the previous chapter we offered you delicious, antioxidant-rich recipes to use, along with the green coffee bean extract, on your new healthy weight-loss plan. In this chapter you're going to get even more strategies to help you get the body you've always wanted without feeling hungry or deprived. Strategies that you can put to work right now to help the weight come off. Strategies that are so simple you'll hardly even know you're trying to lose weight. But lose weight you will! We'll also provide you with shopping tips so you can cruise through the grocery store with a smart plan in place.

HIT YOUR HAPPY WEIGHT WITHOUT PAIN

Losing weight can be hard when you're forced to follow a restrictive food plan. Willpower is a limited resource, and dieting can deplete the resolve of even the most determined person. That's why we've introduced you to a wide variety of foods that are not only good for you, but also delicious and satisfying, precisely so that you won't be deprived while you learn a healthier, high-volume, lower-calorie way of eating. And, most importantly, we taught you about green coffee bean extract, which will accelerate your weight loss.

But we're not done yet! There's plenty more you can do to slim down straightaway—practices and habits that don't take much thought, and take even less willpower. In fact, they don't take any willpower at all. To take true advantage of the power of the green coffee bean extract pill, we've got a few shortcuts to help get you to skinny in no time. Here are a few you can try today:

READ FOOD LABELS

Reading may burn more calories than you think. Not really, but you may be surprised at how it can shave off the pounds. A U.S. National Health Interview Survey examined the eating and shopping habits of twenty-five thousand men and women. An analysis of the data found that on average, women who take the time to look at the nutritional facts on food labels weigh up to nine pounds less than women who don't look at labels. (For a cheat sheet of what label claims mean, see page 116.)

GO NUTS

Adding nuts to your diet could help you lose weight. When Purdue University researchers instructed women to add about two ounces of raw almonds (49 nuts) to their diet daily but gave them no other diet instructions, the women gained no weight, despite the 344-calorie count of the nuts. How is that possible? Researchers theorize the women naturally compensated for most of the extra calories by eating fewer calories throughout the day. Nuts are filling and satisfying.

SHRINK YOUR PLATE

Larger plates can make a serving of food appear smaller, and smaller plates can lead us to believe that same quantity of food is significantly larger. In other words, serving a huge helping of pasta in a big bowl can make us eat more. Or, few stalks of broccoli on a small plate can make us think we've eaten a bunch.

Serve fattening food on smaller plates to trick your sweet tooth into feeling satisfied with less. And dole out healthy food on bigger plates so you'll dish up more.

IMAGINE IT

You don't have to actually eat a fattening food to enjoy it. While you might think that picturing a juicy steak or a hot-fudge sundae would make you crave that food more, a study published in *Science* found that just visualizing yourself eating the food actually dampens your desire to eat it.

People who pictured themselves repeatedly indulging in sweet or salty treats, such as M&Ms and cheese, ended up eating less of the actual foods than people who didn't visualize eating the same foods or thought about them only fleetingly. So instead of immediately digging into that hunk of red velvet cake, picture yourself eating it, bite by bite, and then take a sliver and see if that satisfies you.

DON'T FRATERNIZE WITH FATTIES

Your odds of packing on the pounds increase when you're around people who are overweight. But the converse is true as well—one study found that the spouses of dieters also shed pounds, without even trying. So make sure you're hanging out with friends who are trying to lose weight. If you haven't got any friends who are dieting find an online buddy or join a weight-loss group at a local community center or hospital. Most important, stay away from folks who might discourage your efforts or even sabotage your weight loss.

DON'T BUY IN BULK

That oversize pack of pretzels may save you money, but it will cost you in calories. Researchers at Cornell University found that when people buy huge packages of food, they eat twice as much in the first eight days after they bring them home.

Remember, you can occasionally have anything you want on the green coffee bean extract diet, but you don't want to waste calories munching food you don't really yearn for. Make sure your treats are truly treats—not food you're just eating because it's there. If you don't want to spring for individual serving-size bags of snacks, make your own. Take ten minutes when you get home and divide each pack into snack-size plastic bags for built-in portion control. Two-hundred-calorie snack bags would be about thirty-three almonds, ten pretzel twists, or twenty peanut M&Ms.

EAT MINDFULLY

A University of New Mexico study found that participants who took a mindful eating course lost an average of about 10 pounds over a year. Again, you can have the occasional indulgent treat on the green coffee bean extract diet, but make it count.

Before you take a bite of that rich, velvety chocolate pudding, take a deep breath in through your nose and notice the aroma of the food. Look at the pudding—take note of the deep rich brown color and creamy texture. When you take a spoonful, roll the pudding around your tongue a bit and really experience it. Remember, on the green coffee bean extract diet we want you to enjoy every morsel of food without feeling a morsel of guilt. Take advantage of it!

TURN IN EARLY

Shutting off the lights earlier may keep you away from the junk food. A study published in *Obesity* found that women who go to bed late eat more food at dinner, eat twice as much fast food, and half as many fruits and vegetables than those who turn in earlier.

LABEL LINGO

Comparing products can be difficult with the multitude of label claims. Check out our cheat sheet for decoding help.

- No. A food contains no amount, or a trivial amount of a nutrient.
- Low. Food doesn't easily exceed the dietary guidelines.
- Reduced. Contains at least 25 percent less of a nutrient or of calories than the regular version.
- Lower. Contains 25 percent less of a nutrient or of calories than the regular version.
- Excellent source of. One serving provides 20 percent or more of the daily value for that nutrient.
- Good source of. One serving provides 10 to 19 percent of the daily value for that nutrient.

Biology and environment may factor into the findings. Eating at night when the body is supposed to be sleeping may relate to processing calories differently. Plus, typical go-to late-night snacks are usually unhealthy and high in calories. Make sure you get your seven to eight hours of recommended zzzs: go to sleep and wake up at the same time every day (even on weekends and vacations!), make sure your room is dark, quiet, comfy, and cool, and use your bedroom only for sleep and sex (put away the TV and computer).

HOW TO NAVIGATE THE GROCERY STORE

Sheryl, fifty-two, had great intentions each time she started a new diet. And there were many—the Scarsdale Diet, the Cabbage

Soup Diet, Atkins, South Beach, and the Dukan Diet. But she couldn't stay on any one of those diets for longer than a few weeks because she constantly felt drained and deprived. One of the key secrets to the green coffee bean extract diet is you won't ever feel that way. So many diets leave you feeling hungry and cranky, even weak and fuzzy because you're not putting enough food into your body.

The green coffee bean extract diet puts plenty of food into your body—the difference is that it's good-for-you food, packed with nutrients and filling ingredients so you'll feel alive and energetic, not famished and grouchy. The foods you eat on this diet stimulate your taste buds and satisfy your hunger so you stop eating when you feel sated.

An important component to filling up without filling out is having the right foods on hand at all times. Certain foods can help you torch your metabolism and make the weight fall off, while filling you up and not leaving you hungry. You can find those simple, wholesome foods right in your grocery store. It's not always easy, with the Cocoa Puffs, Devil Dogs, and Milky Way bars calling your name in every other aisle, and when those easy, packaged foods are usually the ones on deep-discount sale. But you can choose foods that make you feel and look great once you know how to look for them. Soon, you won't look twice at those processed, packaged products because you'll love how you feel—and look—without them.

To make sure you end up with bags full of nourishing noshes, it's time to revolutionize your grocery store habits with these pointers in mind:

PLAN AHEAD

Before you even get into the car, plan your meals for the week and create a shopping list. You've got the recipes in the previous pages, so sit down with a pen and a pad of paper and decide what you need. Diana, thirty-two, always felt adrift at the grocery store. She'd wander down this aisle or that, grabbing anything that looked good at the moment. The day she started on the green coffee bean extract diet and decided to shop smarter, she sat down before her grocery store run and took a look through the grocery circular, rifled through her junk drawer for manufacturers' coupons, and put them with a grocery list in her purse. Once at the store, she had a mission in hand.

When you go food shopping, leave the credit cards at home. Instead, estimate how much money you're going to spend and bring just enough cash to pay for what you've planned for, so you won't even have the money to pay for any tempting treats that catch your eye. And eat a healthy snack before you go—some crackers and hummus, or carrots and salsa—so your stomach won't distract you and lead you down the wrong path (aka the chips aisle).

SHOP THE PERIMETER OF THE STORE

That's where you'll find your high-volume fare—veggies, fruit, lean meats, and dairy. Make the produce aisle your first stop. Sure you can pick up the usual—carrots, peas, broccoli, apples, bananas, and strawberries. But don't stop there. Aim to try at least one new fruit or vegetable each week so you won't get bored—try radishes, pomegranates, papaya, or kiwi. And always remember color—baby spinach instead of iceberg lettuce, sweet potatoes instead of plain white ones—for the most nutrition in every bite.

In the meat aisle, choose only lean cuts, ("round" "loin" and "tenderloin" are lighter cuts), including beef, pork, chicken, and turkey. Then pick up some salmon (a healthy fatty fish), shrimp, or other seafood at the fish counter. And choose plenty of low-fat dairy products like yogurt, cheeses, and milk. And don't forget the eggs and whole grains!

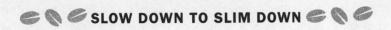

SLOW DOWN TO SLIM DOWN

Want a really simple tip to lose weight? Slow down when you eat. In a study published in the *Journal of the American Dietetic Association,* researchers asked over 1,500 middle-aged women to rank their eating speed based on one of five categories—very slow, slow, medium, relatively fast, or very fast.

What they found was fascinating. For each jump in eating speed—from very slow to slow, or from medium to relatively fast, for example—body weight significantly increased. For example, a five-foot-four woman weighing 165 pounds who ate "very fast" was likely to be almost 20 pounds heavier than her counterpart who ate "very slowly."

To slow down your eating style:

- Take a breath, sip some water, and put down your fork between each bite.
- Dine with a friend, making sure that your mouth is completely empty every time you talk. (A bonus: good manners!)
- Pay close attention to the taste, texture, and smell of every morsel you put in your mouth.
- Put your fork in your nondominant hand, or try eating with chopsticks.

APPROACH THE CENTER AISLES WITH CAUTION

Barbara, thirty-eight, was addicted to packaged foods. At the grocery store she'd head straight to the center aisles. Once she began to read food labels, however, she realized that she was eating far more calories than she thought (not to mention the artificial ingredients and preservatives). She'd always thought that her favorite candy bar was only 120 calories . . . until she real-

CRAVINGS

Sometimes you've got a hankering for something that just won't quit. But your lusts may be satisfied with something less caloric. See if these snack swaps will do the trick.

If you're craving	Candy
Try this instead	Strawberries

If you're craving	Ice cream
Try this instead	Fruit smoothie

If you're craving	Cheesecake
Try this instead	Low-fat Greek yogurt with fruit

If you're craving	Potato chips
Try this instead	Air-popped popcorn

If you're craving	A bagel
Try this instead	A bialy

If you're craving	Bacon
Try this instead	Canadian bacon

If you're craving	French fries
Try this instead	Baked sweet potato fries

If you're craving	Soda
Try this instead	Flavored seltzer

If you're craving	Chocolate
Try this instead	Hot cocoa made with low-fat milk

If you're craving	A margarita
Try this instead	A glass of white wine

If you're craving	Chips and salsa
Try this instead	Chopped jicama with salsa

ized that each bar was two servings! Always look at the serving-size and servings-per-container lines and do the math so you won't make Barbara's mistake. When choosing cereals, look for whole grain and at least five grams of fiber per serving. Frozen fruits and veggies are great, as are canned.

DON'T BE FOOLED BY "NATURAL" LABELING

"Natural" and "organic" are not interchangeable. There's no single set of requirements for products claiming to be natural, but such labels are supposed to be accurate. If, for example, an animal was not fed antibiotics or hormones, then the label should specifically state that. If it just reads "natural" you don't really know what that means. And just because something's organic it doesn't mean it's good for you or won't make you fat. Tricky, we know, but here's why.

The organic label is earned through a certification process, and it means the producer adhered to a strict set of rules and procedures, such as growing vegetables and fruits without any genetically modified seeds, fertilizers made from chemicals or sewage sludge, chemical pesticides or herbicides, and irradiation. Meats must come from animals that were fed only certified organic feed and no by-products of other animals. Better for you? Likely. But organic has nothing to do with fat and calories. Organic foods can still pack on the pounds if you're not aware of what you're eating.

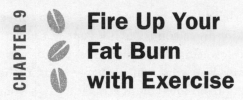

CHAPTER 9

Fire Up Your Fat Burn with Exercise

If you've already begun to take your green coffee bean extract and started following our diet, then you're probably feeling better and lighter already—on the scale and in your head. It feels good to eat a lot of nutritious, delicious foods while losing weight and feeling satisfied, doesn't it? Maybe you have more energy, too, because you're feeding your body food that fuels it, rather than overly refined and processed foods, laden with sugar. You're making good choices for a better long-term lifestyle. And you don't feel deprived, do you?

Put that new-found energy to use and ramp up your weight loss by adding exercise into the mix. We know what you're thinking . . . *Exercise? I don't want to be jumping up and down in spandex pants and leg warmers, sweating to the oldies.*

Don't worry! We've come a long way since the 1980s. There are plenty of fun, exciting ways to move your body to burn calories and boost your metabolism that don't have anything to do with formal exercise.

In this chapter we'll explain why working out is so important to a weight-loss program, and what you can do to get in your requisite activity, even if you don't want to set foot in a gym. Of course, if the exercise bug does bite you, we've got plenty of instruction on more formal exercise plans as well!

MOVE-YOUR-BODY BONUSES

You know that the chlorogenic acid in the green coffee bean extract you're taking has been reducing your gut glucose and fat absorption and lowering your insulin levels to help speed up your metabolism. But what you probably don't realize is that just by switching from low-volume foods to high-volume ones, you've been cutting calories—sometimes drastically—so the weight has been melting off.

Guess what? Adding exercise into the mix can help the weight come off even faster. And exercise has dozens of other benefits as well. Of course, there are the health benefits, including decreased risk of heart attack, stroke, high blood pressure, high cholesterol, and certain types of cancers. And don't forget about the mental benefits of exercise as well. Exercise improves mood, lowers the risk of depression, gives you more energy, promotes better sleep patterns, and even puts an extra spark into your sex life.

Having said all that, we bet you're most interested in how exercise can help you take off those unwanted pounds. So let's take a closer look at what it can do:

EXERCISE HELPS CURB YOUR APPETITE.

Exercise affects the release of two key hunger hormones: ghrelin, produced in the stomach, and peptide tyrosine-tyrosine (PYY), produced in the pancreas. Exercise causes levels of ghrelin (tells the body it's hungry), to drop and PYY levels (tells the body it's full), to increase.

EXERCISE INCREASES CALORIE BURN.

Exercising is a power-punch when it comes to calorie burning. The green coffee extract is helping your body to burn calories, and if you are following our high-volume healthy eating plan, you're also consuming fewer calories. Adding exercise, which also burns calories to your already-reduced calorie plan, will expedite weight loss. But here's the added bonus: exercising doesn't just torch calories while you're working out, it continues to do so all day long.

How? When you lose weight, you can lose muscle along with the fat. Muscle burns more calories than any other tissue in the body. Since exercise helps spare—and build—that calorie-busting muscle, your metabolic rate will be speedier twenty-four/seven.

EXERCISE HELPS IMPROVE SELF-ESTEEM.

Ever hear of the runner's high? Credit endorphins, hormones that are released by the body during exercise that make you feel good. And when you feel good about yourself, sticking with your commitment to weight loss is that much easier. Plus, moving your body can help you feel good about it. Seeing what your body is meant to do—walk, jump, run, dance—can help you see your body as strong and capable, instead of seeing it as a source of torment or torture. Additionally, as you work out, you're getting oxygen-rich blood to your brain, which will give you more energy and make you feel sunnier about life in general.

BURN, BABY, BURN

Joanne hated the thought of exercise. She tried to get herself to the gym a few times a week, but the treadmill was so boring she couldn't stand it more than ten minutes. Even with music on her headset or plugged in to the TV, the monotony of walking and walking to get nowhere just bored her to tears.

You may be just like Joanne; you dread the thought of going to the gym. You've probably scanned this chapter quickly, eager to get on to the next one. You're thinking, *Why can't I just*

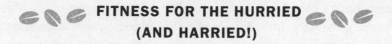

FITNESS FOR THE HURRIED (AND HARRIED!)

These days, everything in our country is designed to save time and energy—remote controls, e-mail, drive-thru, escalators—but these conveniences are also making us fatter. When we think of exercise, we tend to think of going to the gym then getting on with our day (done!). But here's a little secret: the vast majority of total calorie expenditure comes from nonexercise activity thermogenesis (or NEAT), the necessary activity built into the day, such as walking to lunch, cleaning the house, and climbing the stairs.

So, you can sneak calorie-burning activity into your day, and as we well know, the more you use, the less you weigh. Researchers at the Mayo Clinic found that people can increase their NEAT potential by up to 800 calories a day. How can you increase yours? Here are some ideas:

- Walk over to a coworker's desk instead of e-mailing.
- Pace while you talk on the phone.
- Take a walk outside after dinner instead of turning on the TV.
- Ditch the remote and get up every time you want to change the channel. Or do jumping jacks at every commercial.
- Use the bathroom on a different floor, both at work and at home.
- Put your shopping bags in the car each time you make a purchase instead of carrying them with you throughout the mall.
- Do calf raises when waiting in line at the grocery store. Use your cart for balance if you need.
- Skip the drive-thru at the bank, Starbucks, or fast-food restaurant. Always park and get out of your car.
- Meet a friend for a walk instead of a sit-down cup of coffee.
- Whenever possible, stand instead of sit.

The idea is to build movement into your normal routine, ultimately making you an active, not a sedentary, person. Makes sense, right?

let the green coffee bean extract do its job without having to work out at all?

We get it, we really do. But you might want to reconsider just a little. It's clear that everyone stands to benefit from even a small amount of exercise, but if that doesn't convince you to try, here's something else that might help. There are plenty of activities that burn hundreds of calories that don't seem like exercise at all. Just like you're losing weight with your green coffee bean extract without thinking, you could be sizzling calories with exercise and not know it. We're going to introduce you to a couple of activities that are easy, fun, and zap a whole lot of calories. Really!

ZUMBA

Derived from a Colombian word meaning to move fast and have fun, Zumba is like doing an aerobics workout in a South Beach nightclub. It all started when Alberto "Beto" Perez, then an aerobics instructor in Colombia, forgot the music for his class. He dug through his gym bag, came out with some Latin music, and improvised.

That serendipitous class eventually morphed into Zumba, a great, low-impact cardiovascular workout that incorporates the rhythms of the Caribbean, such as salsa, meringue, flamenco, and rumba. The moves are loaded with variations so everyone— from the most limited beginner to the experienced fitness enthusiast—can bust a move. Classes are taught at gyms, libraries, community centers, even schools. Or, if you'd rather do it yourself, try a DVD. For more information, go to zumba.com.

BAR METHOD

You may not be a world-class ballerina, but you can get the same workout as one. Started by former New York City Ballet dancer Mary Helen Bowers, the workout integrates the fat-burning format of interval training, muscle-shaping technique of isometrics, elongating principles of dance conditioning, and the science of physical therapy, to provide even the least graceful among us the techniques to quickly build and maintain the beauty and strength of a ballet dancer's form.

There are now more than sixty-five Bar Method studios across the country and Canada, as well as a DVD workout. Visit barmethod.com for more information.

CARDIO KICKBOXING

Ever wanted to kick the you-know-what out of someone? In kickboxing classes, you can pretend to do just that! Often a mix of martial arts and boxing, cardio kickboxing is an intense, total-body, stress-relieving workout. Classes vary—some use boxing equipment like bags, gloves, and jump ropes, some use hand weights, and others use nothing at all. But all lead you through a combination of jabs, hooks, uppercuts, and kicks that help improve your balance, coordination, strength, and of course, burn oodles of calories.

AERIAL YOGA

Think yoga's a funky workout? How about yoga done in a suspended hammock? AntiGravity Yoga was first developed by Christopher Harrison, a former aerial acrobat and gymnast. It blends traditional yoga with acrobatics, gymnastics, Pilates, and calisthenics and truly allows you to explore the poses from a whole new perspective.

The weightless poses can be used to strengthen the core as well as relieve aching joints and stretch tight muscles. The supportive equipment helps you feel confident and experience less joint compression when performing inversion poses like handstand. At the same time, the stretchy material pushes you to find greater depth and range of movement.

See if a class is available near you at www.antigravityyoga.com, or you can get an inversion swing for your own home.

URBAN REBOUNDING

If you ever went to summer camp, you probably loved every minute on the trampoline. Who says you can't do it as an adult and torch calories at the same time? Trampoline classes are jumping up all across the country. With the trampoline you get all the benefits of a high-intensity workout, but the tramp's bounce takes the pressure off your back and joints.

Not only will you be melting away the fat and inches, you'll also strengthen every muscle in your body (including your core) and improve balance and coordination. Urban rebounding classes are taught across the country, as well as through an in-home, independent workout.

WHY LONGER ISN'T ALWAYS BETTER

The number-one reason people give for not exercising is that they don't have enough time. And we know that one reason you chose the green coffee bean extract diet is because you want to lose weight in the easiest way possible. But the no-time excuse won't cut it in this plan. Because we're here to tell you that exercising too hard or for too long is counterproductive. Extended endurance training is not the best way to improve your stamina and strength nor is it the best way to burn fat and calories. Plus, it takes up your valuable time and increases your risk of injury.

The body is highly adaptive, and when you challenge it again and again in the same way, it will adjust to meet the challenge with less effort. So over time, long duration exercise will actually encourage your heart, lungs, and muscles to expend less energy during long bouts of activity. Instead of burning *more* calories, the body becomes more efficient and actually burns *fewer*.

WANT TO BURN 100 CALORIES? HERE ARE 12 EASY WAYS TO DO IT.

- Dance for 20 minutes
- Vacuum for 25 minutes
- Pull weeds for 20 minutes
- Rake for 40 minutes
- Mow the lawn for 20 minutes
- Jog for 10 minutes
- Iron clothes for 40 minutes
- Wash your car for 30 minutes
- Bowl for 30 minutes
- Jump rope for 10 minutes
- Organize your closet for 35 minutes
- Plant flowers for 20 minutes

So what's the answer? Switch it up! The most effective way to zap calories with exercise is to do something different all the time, so your body never gets too good at any one thing. Mix up the activities you do every day—not only does that keep your body from adapting, it also keeps you from getting bored.

INTERVAL INSTRUCTION

Another option to get around your body's ability to adapt is an innovative method of training, called interval training. Intervals can help maximize your calorie and fat burn and increase the strength and aerobic capacity of your heart and lungs. Best of all, interval workouts take only twenty to thirty minutes a day.

With interval training, you alternate short bursts of intense exertion with short periods of recovery, rather than exercise for

WALK THIS WAY

If walking's your workout choice, you're probably not giving a thought to how you walk. But just like any exercise, walking requires proper form. How to do it: Think of the crown of your head reaching toward the ceiling. Your shoulders should be back and down, your arms bent naturally at the elbow. Your pelvis should be tucked under your torso and stomach pulled in tight. Feet should go heel, ball, toe, heel, ball, toe.

If you want to pick up speed, don't take bigger steps. Instead, concentrate on driving your elbows back faster, and your feet will naturally follow. Don't look down, which will strain your neck and back. Instead, look fifteen to twenty feet ahead of you, keeping your chin level with the ground.

long periods of time. What's incredible is that with interval training, you not only burn calories during the time you're exercising, you also step up your fat-burning metabolism in the hours *following* exercise.

Adding interval training to any workout is easy. Some activities—tennis and racquet ball, for instance—have built in intervals. Other activities—like walking, running, and biking—can easily be adapted as an interval-training workout. Here's how: Begin by warming up at a moderate pace for five minutes to get the blood pumping throughout your body. (See page 128 for more information on warming up and cooling down.) When you feel warm and your heartbeat and breathing are slightly accelerated, you're ready to roll.

Alternate two minute of hard-as-you-can walking, sprinting, biking, swimming (or whatever activity you're doing), with one to two minutes of recovery. In other words, walk, run, bike, or swim absolutely as hard or as fast as you can, but just for two short minutes. Then, back off the pace and recover for one to two minutes. For your recovery intervals you want to slow down enough to catch your breath, but keep moving. By the end of your recovery interval, you should be ready for another sprint.

Keep going, alternating sprint and recovery intervals for a total of twenty minutes. Your workout will be finished before you even realize you've broken a sweat. If you don't want to think too hard about it, see if your treadmill, stationary bikes, stair stepper, etc., has a preprogrammed interval-training setting, which changes the speed, resistance, or incline of the machine for you. Many do.

Don't get too hung up on the exact time you're doing everything. The Swedish refer to intervals as *fartlek* training. Translation: speed play. Take your cue from the Swedish and play with your workout. Have fun with it. Sometimes speed up quickly then take awhile to slow down. For the next interval, slowly speed up until you start to become breathless and then slow down gradually. The most important rule is to have fun—and just keep your body moving!

LIFT TO LOSE

In addition to working your heart, you want to also engage your muscles with free weights or machines, or any other form of resistance, such as weighted cuffs, rubber resistance bands, or tubes. You can even use the weight of your own body, with push-ups, chin-ups, lunges, and dips. We know what you're thinking: *Hey, I don't want to look like a body builder.* We can assure you, there's little chance of that. Super-buff women spend hours lifting very heavy weights, and they're usually also taking large amounts of body-building supplements. Big muscles don't develop by accident—it takes a lot of work to make them look that way.

But you need to utilize your muscles because, when done

correctly, strength training will tighten and sculpt the muscles of your body and burn away excess body fat. And contrary to what you might think, strength training will not make you bigger—it will actually make you smaller, shapelier, and fit.

You've heard that muscle weighs more than fat, right? That's not really the truth—a pound of muscle weighs the same exact pound as that pound of fat. What *is* true, though, is that a pound of muscle takes up much less space than a pound of fat. So taking off a pound of fat and putting on a pound of muscle will make you smaller—and fit into those skinny jeans easier!

RESISTANCE TRAINING THE RIGHT WAY

You're busy, we know. But the good news is that when you do resistance training the right way, you don't need a whole lot of time. One set of eight to ten repetitions is all you need to get a great workout, and you can easily work all the major muscles in the body in about twenty minutes. And while you should try to get some sort of aerobic activity at least five or six days a week, you can get the benefits of resistance training in only two sessions a week. (Take at least one day off between sessions.)

So, to do your resistance training right, and in the most time-efficient way, you have to challenge your muscles in a very specific way. If you can repeat any strength-training exercise more than twelve times, you're not working hard enough. Step up the resistance until you find that the ninth or tenth repetition is difficult to complete. To increase the difficulty without increasing the resistance, you can also increase "time under tension" by slowing your movements down and not allowing the muscles to relax in between repetitions.

If you've never done strength training, invest in a few sessions with a personal trainer to learn how to do it correctly. The better your form, the better your results will be and the lower your risk of injury.

Ironically, when you use good form, you will probably need

less weight to fatigue the muscle, because proper form will more effectively isolate the muscle you're working. And you'll get more benefit from lifting slightly less weight with good form than you will from lifting more weight with poor form. Ultimately, the amount of resistance doesn't matter. What matters is that the (correct) muscle is fatigued when you finish your set.

WARMING UP AND COOLING DOWN

The warm-up and cool-down of any exercise program are not unlike going to the dentist; you know you have to do it, but you skip it as much as possible. But just like going to the dentist is a must, easing into your workout beforehand, and cooling down afterward are necessities, too. Slowly raising your core temperature and getting extra blood and oxygen to the heart and muscles give your body a chance to adjust and help reduce the risk of injury. Cooling down afterward helps to gradually reduce the temperature of all your muscles, reducing stiffness and soreness.

So, whatever workout you're doing, take a few minutes at the beginning to start in low gear. If you're going for a walk, walk slowly for a few minutes before you pick up the pace. In the pool, do a few easy laps before picking up the tempo. When weight training, move your body through the movement patterns you'll do during the exercises before you start with the weights.

At the end of your workout, slow down the speed and intensity gradually to give your body time to recover. And do some easy stretches to help improve performance and decrease your risk of injury.

Try the following stretch routine. Do each stretch three to five times on both sides, and hold for about ten to thirty seconds. Never bounce. Instead, breathe into the move and feel your body relaxing. Stretching should feel good, not painful.

1. Take one big step back, bend your front knee slightly and press your back heel down to the floor until you feel

a release in your calf. Bring your legs together and repeat on the other side.

2. Place the heel of one foot in front of you, bend the other knee slightly and push your tush back in the opposite direction to stretch your hamstrings. Place your hands on your upper thighs or your hips for balance. Bring your feet back to the center and repeat on the other side.

3. Bend your right knee and bring your right heel up toward your buttocks, holding your ankle with your right hand (grab something for balance if necessary). Try to keep your knees aligned and feel the stretch in the front of your thigh. Press your pelvis forward to get an additional stretch in the hip area. Put your foot down then repeat on the other side.

4. Reach up straight and tall and lace your fingers together, stretching upward. Then take your right arm and reach it toward the left side, stretching the entire right side of the body. Repeat toward the other side.

CHAPTER 10

Frequent Fumbles

Jackie, thirty-three, was determined to lose weight. She'd tried diets before but never lost the last 10 pounds she had put on with her second baby. She went to the grocery store and bought the requisite carrots and celery. And she threw out all the junk food in the house. She thought, *If I'm going to do this, I'm going to go all out.*

She ate almost nothing for seven straight days and worked up a sweat for two hours every day. When she stepped on the scale, she couldn't wait to see the huge drop she expected. Instead, she was horrified. She'd lost a mere quarter of a pound. Why? Jackie fell prey to one of the biggest diet mistakes there is: She went in gung ho, doing too much too soon, and she cut out too many calories.

How on earth could cutting too many calories be a mistake, you might ask. Read on, and you'll find out the somewhat surprising explanation below when we talk about the weight-loss blunder many people make: thinking you have to starve to lose weight.

When people begin a diet, they have very high hopes. Many dive in head first, without truly thinking through a plan. They believe if they start the diet with good intentions, the weight will come off.

Unfortunately, often the very practices you think are the most helpful are the ones that stop you from losing weight. This is why the green coffee bean extract diet is so effective; good intentions are really all you need if you're taking the supplement. Without making any drastic changes, the weight will come off.

However, even with this simple premise—eat when you're hungry, focus on high-volume foods, and take your green coffee bean extract as directed—you're bound to make mistakes. In this chapter, we'll show you some of the most common setbacks and errors. We'll show you why you may not be losing weight, and what you can do to turn those habits around.

We'll also look at some of the biggest hurdles that are working against you and your plan, factors such as your job, your kids, or even your spouse. Then, after we take a look at all those potential roadblocks, we get you back on track to lose weight, feel satisfied, and look great.

WHY YOUR WAISTLINE ISN'T WHITTLING

It's not too hard to figure out why many dieters fail over and over again. Even on the most straightforward diet like the one in this book, it doesn't take much to veer off course. Here are some oft-repeated blunders that may be the culprits to keeping you corpulent.

With just a little adjustment and a willingness to try something different, we're confident that the green coffee bean extract diet will help you achieve the goals that have eluded you for so long. Remember, it's not about denying yourself to get skinny short-term, but about eating a lot of health-supporting, tasty foods that will aid in your long-term goal of staying slim.

YOU THINK YOU HAVE TO STARVE TO LOSE WEIGHT.

With spring in the air, Caitlin needed to lose the 15 pounds she'd gained over the winter. So she cut down her food intake to almost nothing. She ate a tiny bowl of cereal in the morning, a salad for lunch, and some plain grilled chicken for dinner. *What gives?* she thought as she stepped on the scale and hadn't lost an ounce.

When people go on diets, they think they have to slash portion sizes down to practically nothing. *If I'm not hungry, I couldn't possibly be losing weight,* they think. But anything that smacks of deprivation is going to wind up kicking you in the butt. Because, as we've said many times throughout this book, the more restricted you feel, the more likely you are to go off the deep end later.

Plus, nobody's told your body that you've chosen not to eat, so it goes into starvation mode, adapting to your lower food intake in order to stop from wasting away. Remember Jackie? This is exactly why she stopped losing weight. Our bodies are incredible specimens, and this, as experts call it, "starvation response" is probably left over from the caveman days. Back then, man didn't know when his next meal was coming, so if the caveman's body continued to burn calories at a steady rate when buffalo meat ran short, he'd soon run out of fuel. Not a good thing for a caveman.

Instead, when food ran low, he began to burn the calories he did take in more efficiently. In the same way, when you're on a diet, the body senses that sustenance is in short supply and it holds on to what it has for dear life.

The whole point of the green coffee bean extract diet is that you can eat a ton of food and still lose weight. Think high volume: for the calories in one piece of chocolate cake, you could have ten chocolate Tootsie Pops, two pints of chocolate sorbet, forty-four dried apricot halves, twenty-eight butterscotch candies, or two whole pineapples. No need to starve when you're eating in a high-volume way!

YOU'RE DOING TOO MUCH TOO SOON.

Sheri, forty-four, went into every diet like gangbusters. She changed all her eating patterns and exercised like crazy. And then, after a week of starvation and aching muscles, she'd say, "The hell with this," and go off the diet. Big, grand changes are a surefire way to fail because all the restrictions and rules to remember are overwhelming.

It doesn't have to be like that when you're on the green coffee bean extract diet. Rather than implement radical change, now is a good time to explore those habits that caused you to gain weight in the first place. Don't try to tackle them all at once; it will be more manageable to take on one at a time.

Perhaps you're one of those people who eats a whole bag of potato chips in front of the television. Vow to eat only in the dining room. When you've conquered that, promise yourself you'll eat a yogurt and a few pretzels instead of that Snickers bar for your afternoon work breaks. Or that you'll pack healthy snacks so you won't feel the urge to raid the vending machine. And so on.

YOU FEEL GUILTY WHEN YOU "CHEAT."

Marni, thirty-eight, had a life-long obsession with ice cream. She'd tell herself she'd eat, "just a spoonful," and then she couldn't stop until the entire pint of Rocky Road was gone. Or the gallon. And then she'd feel guilty and shameful, vowing to starve herself as punishment for the foreseeable future.

The more "forbidden" a food is, the more you'll want it. So, instead of swearing off all your favorite foods, allow yourself to have them. Remember, you've got the power of green coffee bean extract in your corner. It's okay to allow yourself some treats. And when you stop feeling guilty about eating your favorite foods, they'll no longer have that unhealthy grip over you. Enjoy the occasional slice of pizza outright, and you won't feel the need to scarf down the entire pie in shame.

YOU SKIP BREAKFAST.

Carly, twenty-four, never ate breakfast. A morning meal didn't thrill her, and she figured that saving those calories would help her lose weight. Not so much. No matter how tempting it is to bump breakfast off your to-do list, studies show that you absolutely must eat it in order to lose weight. In fact, almost 80 percent of the people who successfully lose weight and keep it off eat breakfast every day according to the National Weight Control Registry, a database of more than five thousand people who have lost and kept off more than 30 pounds.

Breakfast is critical to kick-start your metabolism after a night of not eating. And morning munching can reduce your hunger later in the day, making it easier to avoid binging. When you buck breakfast, you may feel famished later, making it nearly impossible to choose healthy fare. Your body can only store a limited amount of glucose—the body's main source of energy. If you don't replenish your glucose stores after an evening's fast, blood sugar begins to plummet, sending stronger and stronger messages to the brain that it needs food STAT.

Even if you don't have time to sit down for a long meal, a smoothie takes no time at all (see recipe on page 74). Prep the ingredients the night before so all you need to do is whip it up in the blender and put it in a to-go cup.

YOU'RE SUPER FRIGHTENED OF FAT . . .

It sounds counterintuitive, but you actually need fat *in* your body to lose it *on* your body. We all need some fat, both to feel full and to stay full longer. Fat is a concentrated source of energy that takes longer to digest than either protein or carbs, keeping you feeling fuller longer. While saturated fats, such as butter, red meats, and cheeses are high-density and it's best to cut back on them as much as you can, good fats from fatty fish (salmon, trout, and mackerel), avocados, walnuts, olive oil, and flaxseed can keep you from overeating overall. Remember one of the main rules of the green coffee bean extract diet: replace bad fats with good!

AND YOU SEE A FAT-FREE LABEL AS A LICENSE TO PIG OUT.

Michelle, thirty-six, couldn't understand why she wasn't losing weight. She started her day eating cereal with fat-free milk, ate nothing but salads at lunch and snacked on fat-free candy all day. After a healthy dinner she'd snuggle up to a big hunk of fat-free cheesecake each night. One slice usually didn't take the edge off, so she'd go back for another. And another. *It doesn't matter,* she thought, *because it's fat-free.*

Our nation's fear of fat has triggered a proliferation of processed low-fat and no-fat products. But you can be on a zero-fat diet and still gain weight. When you scarf down those fat-free products, you usually end up taking in more calories than you would if you were eating something you deemed fattening. Sometimes the product contains more sugar or salt to make it taste better; other times, you just won't find the bland flavor satisfying, so you'll end up eating more than you should in order to get your fix. And all those excess calories, whether from a carbohydrate, protein, or fat, end up as fat on the body.

Instead of thinking solely about the fat grams in a product, think about the number of calories and portion size as well. Sometimes you actually might do better taking a sliver of the most fattening (and tasty!) chocolate cake than taking a slab of the fat-free version. Then you're not denying yourself what you *really* want (an important premise of the green coffee bean extract diet!), and you'll satisfy that craving with *one* reasonable portion. You'll still be on track with your healthy eating plan.

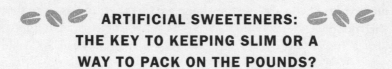

ARTIFICIAL SWEETENERS: THE KEY TO KEEPING SLIM OR A WAY TO PACK ON THE POUNDS?

Sugar substitutes seem like they could be the magic potion for weight loss. They pack a hundred times more sweetening punch than table sugar, so you only need a dash to get that sweet taste, potentially saving hundreds of calories a day. But they may, in fact, backfire when it comes to weight loss.

One study published in *Obesity* found that participants who drank more than twenty-one diet drinks per week were twice as likely to become overweight as people who didn't down the synthetic sweet stuff. Artificial sweeteners may stoke your sweet tooth and set off cravings that lead you to binge on high-calorie foods later. So, your best bet is to use sugar substitutes in moderation, and focus mostly on natural, nutritious, high-volume foods like fruits, vegetables, lean meats, and whole grains. Remember, a once-in-a-while treat of something with *real* sugar will satisfy you much more than a whole lot of something with sugar substitute.

YOU'RE RELYING TOO MUCH ON THE SCALE.

Although seeing the numbers drop on the scale can be encouraging, seeing them stay the same can be frustrating. But weight is not the sole measurement of how you're doing on a diet. Remember in the previous chapter when we talked about how muscle is denser than fat, so it takes up less space on your body? That means that although you may not be seeing the numbers on the scale go down, if you're following our high-volume food plan, taking your green coffee bean extract, and exercising, you're probably getting tighter and buffer and looking a whole lot better.

And if you're a woman, you know that your weight can fluctuate during your menstrual cycle (hello bloat!). If you've splurged on something salty the night before, you could be retaining water. Instead of obsessing over the scale, use a tape measure to check your shrinking waistline. Or use a pair of skinny jeans as a gauge of how slim you're getting.

HOW TO OVERCOME ANY OBSTACLE

Even if you're doing all the right things, there may be people or places along your journey to a new, slimmer you that get in your way. Let's take a look at some of the greatest stumbling blocks you might face on this voyage. In this section, we'll also offer you some pointers to power through even the most challenging times when you think you can't keep going. Because on the green coffee bean extract diet, unlike any other, you really can.

YOUR CHILDREN

Being a mom is tough enough. But being a mom on a diet? Nearly impossible. Sandy, forty, felt like a short-order cook when it came to planning meals. Her daughter wanted steak, her older son wanted a hamburger, and her little one wanted macaroni and cheese. If that's not enough, she also had to play chauffeur, homework assistant, and nurse. No wonder she had neither the time nor the energy to pay attention to what she ate. But Sandy's bites of mac and cheese and burgers added up, and she became seriously overweight.

She decided to try the green coffee bean extract diet and put a few other strategies into place. She vowed to eat only food that came from her own bowl, plate, or cup. And she planned ahead, making a big vat of vegetarian chili and a few broth-based soups on Sunday night to freeze for dinners during the rest of the week. She prepped delicious morning frittatas to freeze as well. She stashed some healthy snacks—almonds and raisins—in the car and at her desk drawer at work. And she used her kids to her advantage, jumping rope with them, playing tag, and going swimming. In just three months, Sandy took off 20 pounds.

YOUR FRIENDS

While it would be nice for all your friends to come together and sing the Kumbaya weight-loss theme song, the reality is that some friends will feel resentful of your new healthy eating strategy and some might even try to sabotage your successes. Losing weight can mean that something you may once have had in common with your friends is now gone. It will take some time for everyone to get used to your new way of life.

Make sure to include your friends in the transition—sign up for a run/walk with a buddy or invite her to check out a new healthy restaurant you've found. Or, instead of sharing a meal, ask her to meet you for a walk around the block or a movie. You'll bring the air-popped popcorn!

YOUR SPOUSE

It's tough when you've finally got the kids in bed and you can't wait to finally put your feet up and watch a little *Downton Abbey,* and then whammo, your husband sits down next to you, munching on a bag of chips. Although spouses say they'll be supportive, the reality is that they rarely actually give you what you need when you're trying to lose weight.

With your husband comfortably crunching on his chips, resist the urge to find the nearest sledgehammer and instead, tell him how you feel. "Honey, I love spending time with you but I'm trying to eat more healthfully. Could you eat the chips (quietly!) in the other room?" Or suggest that you both munch on a healthy snack together. Try one of these: three cups air-popped pop-corn, two cups frozen grapes or berries, single-size serving cin-namon soy chips, or two squares of dark chocolate. Who knows, maybe he'll join you on the green coffee bean extract diet and you'll both feel better!

YOUR TRAVEL SCHEDULE

Traveling, whether it's for business or pleasure, can make even the best dieter's intentions go kafluey. When Katie, twenty-nine, landed a new job that forced her to travel at least three times per month, eating at airports and out with clients made taking off those extra 10 pounds seem impossible. Within a year, not only had she not reached her goal of losing 10 pounds, she actually gained another 15 pounds.

She decided to try the green coffee bean extract diet and resisted the urge to scarf down a Cinnabon in every airport. In-stead, she used her time at the airport to get in some exercise—walking around and window shopping—and she stopped using the moving walkways and escalators. She also made it a rule never to ditch breakfast—no matter how strapped for time she was—so she didn't end up ravenous later in the day. Within a month she'd lost 5 pounds, and the rest of the weight slid off easily.

COCKTAIL PARTIES

Even the best of dieters cave to cocktail party pressure. Free drinks and delicious finger foods displayed on trays for the taking—who can resist?

You can! Never go to a party hungry—have a light snack with a bit of protein beforehand. Broth-based soup or some whole-wheat crackers with hummus are some good options. When you get to the party, vow to work yourself around the room at least once before you head toward the buffet table.

When loading your plate, try a fifty-fifty rule—take everything you want, no matter how fattening it is, but take an equal amount of healthy foods, too; if you want seconds, go for it—just make sure you balance the plate again. And the fifty-fifty rule applies to drinks, too. For every alcoholic beverage you imbibe, you should also have a big glass of sparkling water.

DINING OUT

Lots of people use dinner out as a license to go crazy. While you're taking the green coffee bean extract, it's okay to diverge from your diet every once in a while, but try not to go completely off the rails. The more you stick with your diet strategies, the quicker the weight will come off.

Ask for a quiet table away from the action—the more distractions around you (by a window or in front of a television), the more you can shovel in your mouth without thinking. Once seated, scan the menu. Be aware of anything too descriptive like "succulent," "velvety," or "juicy" that can make you order more. Request that your food be grilled, steamed, or broiled instead of sautéed or fried. And order a lunch portion, even at dinner. Tempted by dessert? Treat yourself to three forkfuls and you may be satisfied and say *finis*.

CHAPTER 11

Getting Past the Plateau

Mary, forty-nine, followed the green coffee bean extract diet and took off 15 pounds. She was thrilled when all her friends, and even the folks at her local grocery store, complimented her on how great she looked. Mary was excited to step on the scale every Friday morning to see her progress. With only 5 pounds to go, she continued with her plan and downed her green coffee bean extract before each meal. When Friday rolled around, she stepped on the scale, looked down, and instead of the two-pound drop she usually saw, her weight was the same as it was the week before. She figured this was a fluke and kept going. But the next week, it seemed like the scale was stuck again. Mary was upset, but continued to follow the plan. When she stepped on the scale the next Friday and she'd only dropped a half a pound, she knew something was amiss.

Mary had hit what experts call a plateau—a phase when the scale needle won't budge even though there's still some weight to be lost. Since those last fat cells have been there the longest, they're going to be the toughest to lose. Mary's not the only dieter who's had this experience. You likely will, too, if you haven't already.

At the point of plateau, many throw in the diet towel disgusted and feeling like failures. Others keep trying, doing what they've been doing all along, hoping something will eventually give. Too often, the only thing these dieters are left with is the belief that nothing works.

Don't despair! You're in this for the long haul, remember? The green coffee bean extract diet is about eating delicious foods, feeling sated, and creating healthier habits that will sustain you for a lifetime. We will get you where you want to be. In this chapter we're going to explore why the dreaded plateau happens, and we'll give you strategies on what you can do to get the weight coming off once again.

WHY DOES THE SCALE STALL?

Most diets follow a pretty typical pattern. The first week or so is the most fun—the weight seems to slide off, almost too easily—though in reality, it's mostly water weight that's being shed. As you cut calories, your body releases its stores of glycogen, a type of carbohydrate found in the muscles and liver. Glycogen holds on to water, so when glycogen is burned for energy, it releases water.

As you stick to your green coffee bean extract diet, your body loses fat and muscle mass; the less fat and muscle mass you have, the slower your basal metabolic rate will be. Your basal metabolic rate is the number of calories you burn doing absolutely nothing, and it accounts for the majority of calories you burn every day. In other words, at your thinner weight, you're burning fewer calories doing the same activities than you did at your heavier weight.

It's a cruel irony of dieting; although you may look and feel a whole lot better, at your new weight, calories eaten now equal calories burned. So doing what you've been doing up until now will keep you at your current weight, but won't work to take off any more weight.

Put your hands in the air and back away from the chocolate cake! Take a deep breath and don't get so frustrated that you revert back to your old habits. Remember, the green coffee bean extract diet is about developing healthier habits and attitudes, while relishing food that tastes good and is good for you. And this diet is about developing skills to manage the most challenging moments. So, let's take a look at some strategies you can use to get that scale to move downward again.

GET BACK TO THE BASICS

When you're closest to your goal, you may unwittingly get a little sloppy. You may be taking a few bites of your daughter's macaroni and cheese or sneaking more than one high-calorie treat every day. Why don't you take a few days to record everything you put in your mouth? That means every BLT (bite, lick, and taste!). In your food diary, include the times of day you're eating, as well as what you're feeling before and after you ate, to spot any problem times or emotions that may be causing you to binge. Once you recognize a problem, it will be easier to tackle.

You could also try weighing your food for a bit. We're not talking about weeks at a time, but just for a few days, to give yourself a more accurate picture of how many calories you're truly consuming. A key reason for a weight loss plateau is eating more than you think. It's easy for portion sizes to creep up, and before you know it, you end up eating way more than you should. Backsliding by even an extra 200 calories a day could be what's slowing your weight loss.

ADD SOME FAT

It might sound counterintuitive—not to mention counterproductive—but fat is actually a dietary necessity. (We talked about this in the previous chapter.) A concentrated source of energy, fat helps you feel fuller longer. Two slices of avocado on your sandwich or a handful of nuts may keep you from overeating at the next meal—and keep you on the losing track. And as we've mentioned before, don't fall for the fat-free processed food fraud; many such products are actually higher in calories than their full-fat counterparts—and you might scarf down two or three times the serving size to satisfy your craving.

STOP THE SELF-SABOTAGE

Sometimes the biggest obstacle to losing those last few pounds is your own mind. People often blame all sorts of personal issues on their weight. Yet if the weight were no longer there, then they'd have to deal directly with the problems they've tried so long and hard to avoid.

Try to identify anything about reaching your goal weight that makes you anxious. Are you frightened of attention—whether it's positive or negative? If so, imagine what you would say if someone said you looked great. Or, if you're unsure of how others will react, picture yourself in a room full of people who haven't seen you in a long time. In your visualization, imagine yourself smiling, holding your head up, and making eye contact. By practicing mentally, you're far more likely to actually achieve your goal, because you'll feel prepared.

DON'T CUT FOOD, REDISTRIBUTE IT

Determine when you tend to eat your biggest meal. If it's during the evening hours, rethink your timing. Why fuel yourself with more calories when you're actually slowing down for the day? Instead, try eating about the same amount of food, but take in more food earlier in the day and taper off at night. Chances are, by consuming more early on, you'll have more energy and you'll move even more—burning more calories—during the day. Or, try eating the same amount of food per week, but make some days heavier in calories than others. Just by switching things up, you may kick-start your metabolism back into high gear.

EAT SMALLER MEALS MORE OFTEN

How often you eat may not matter (from a metabolic standpoint) in terms of your body's ability to burn calories, but in terms of how satisfied you feel, it can make a big difference. Eating at regular intervals helps keep blood sugar levels up, which makes it easier to stick to your eating plan. Eat five to six mini meals of complex carbohydrates (fruits and veggies) with a small amount of protein and fat. The carbs will get used quickly for energy, while the protein and fat, which are digested more slowly, will give you energy for the long term.

LIFT A FEW POUNDS TO DROP A FEW POUNDS

We discussed exercise and the importance of resistance exercise in chapter 9, but have you been following our advice? Many people get cardio happy and skip weight training when they're exercising. After all, lifting weights isn't all that exciting and it doesn't give you that same immediate rush as running or Zumba class. But resistance training is crucial for you to take off those last few pounds. Remember, muscle uses more calories to maintain itself than other body tissue—so even when you're reading *50 Shades of Grey*, the more muscle you have throughout your body, the more calories you'll be burning.

If nothing else, weight training allows you to keep exercising once you're too pooped to stay on the treadmill. If you haven't yet been weight training, focus your strength work on the waist down. The lower body contains more muscle mass than the upper body, so you'll be working more muscle fibers and burning more calories per workout session. Compound exercises—moves that involve more than one joint, such as squats, lunges, and leg presses—also activate more total muscle, increasing both calorie burn and strength.

Experiment with using free weights rather than exercise machines. Weight machines isolate a joint, thus working a single muscle or muscle group, while free weights enlist other muscles throughout the body to maintain stability, form, and alignment. More muscles working equals more calories burned.

BECOME A CALORIE WASTER

Remember, the vast majority of your total calorie expenditure comes from daily activities. Expand your definition of exercise beyond what you do in sneakers and sweats. Look for opportunities to use energy in a world that's increasingly designed to conserve it. Run out for lunch instead of ordering in, take extra trips to the car and back, and in general, squander your steps.

REARRANGE YOUR REFRIGERATOR

Eating those high-volume fruits and veggies can help you keep trim, but unfortunately, many of us throw out more than we eat. In fact, produce makes up about a quarter of the food you trash every day. Stashing the good stuff in produce drawers usually means you forget about it and it goes bad before you've gotten a chance to eat it. To make sure that fruits and vegetables remain a mainstay of your diet, wash and cut them up as soon as you get home from the supermarket and store everything in airtight containers, on eye-level shelves. Keep a fruit bowl on the counter with apples, pears, bananas, or mangos. And don't buy more than a week's worth of produce at a time.

RELAX AND RIDE IT OUT

Sometimes what you think is a plateau really isn't one at all. If you don't lose weight over the course of one week, don't panic. Maybe you're premenstrual or ate a particularly salty meal the night before and your body is retaining water. Or you may have

PUT ON A PEDOMETER

Even if you're exercising a few times a week, you can up your activity level and burn more calories by simply wearing a pedometer, a device that counts the number of steps you take. Clip it to your pants first thing in the morning to get your baseline and add 15 percent to that number for the next week or two. For each following week, increase it by another 15 percent. Make it a point to be more active throughout the day—pace when you talk on the phone, use the stairs instead of the elevator, and take the dog on an extra walk. Your ultimate goal: at least ten thousand steps every day.

weighed yourself incorrectly. Give yourself a few weeks before you declare a plateau. Meanwhile, look to other measures of success—a smaller clothing size, a feeling of greater energy, a change in body measurements—to keep you going until that needle inches down again.

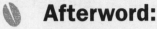
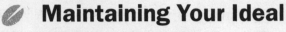
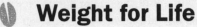

Afterword: Maintaining Your Ideal Weight for Life

The green coffee bean extract diet has given you an arsenal of tools to put you on the fast track to easy, deprivation-free weight loss. Whether you've lost 5 pounds or 50, you're going to want to keep those pounds gone for good.

Once you've reached your goal, you no longer have to take the supplement. However, you should continue the diet and exercise plan for life. The menu plans and suggestions we've given you are things you can continue for years to come, without any drama or fuss.

Keep the book nearby as a reference. Just in case the weight begins to creep back, take your green coffee bean extract again, skim through these pages, and the weight should fall back off. Remember, the diet plan we've given you is one that can keep you healthy and happy for life. So why eat any other way?